FREEDOM

from

DIGESTIVE
DISTRESS

FREEDOM

from

DIGESTIVE DISTRESS

MEDICINE-FREE RELIEF
From Heartburn, Gas, Bloating, and Irritable Bowel Syndrome

GARY GITNICK, M.D.

Chief, Division of Digestive Diseases, UCLA School of Medicine

WITH KAREN COOKSEY

Produced by The Philip Lief Group, Inc.

THREE RIVERS PRESS • NEW YORK

Published by Three Rivers Press, New York, New York.
Member of the Crown Publishing Group.

Random House, Inc. New York, Toronto, London, Sydney,
Auckland www.randomhouse.com

THREE RIVERS PRESS is a registered trademark
and the Three Rivers Press colophon is a trademark of
Random House, Inc.

Printed in the United States of America
Design by Rhea Braunstein

Library of Congress Cataloging-in-Publication Data
Gitnick, Gary L.
Freedom from digestive distress : medicine-free relief from
heartburn, gas, bloating, and irritable bowel syndrome /
Gary Gitnick, with Karen Cooksey.
p. cm.
Includes index.
1. Indigestion—Popular works.   I. Cooksey, Karen.   II. Title.
RC827.G55   2000
616.3'32—dc21
00-037724

ISBN 0-812-93262-5 (pbk.)

10   9   8   7   6   5   4   3   2   1

First Edition

AUTHOR'S NOTE

No book, including this one, can ever substitute for a doctor's visit. I hope that you'll want to share a copy of this book with your physician so that he or she can work more effectively with you to help you overcome your digestive distress. I've learned so much from my patients over the years and I hope that what I've written here will both help you unlock the secrets of your own ailment and encourage your doctor to spread the word that a take-charge attitude and proper self-care can work wonders. Good luck and good health to you.

CONTENTS

....

ACKNOWLEDGMENTS

....

I am indebted to Susan Dashe for her dedicated effort in helping to put together this manuscript, as well as to Jamie Saxon of The Philip Lief Group for her faithful pursuit of excellence and her efficient management of the book development and, to Betsy Rapoport of Three Rivers Press for her insightful editorial advice and decisions.

Finally, all of my books have been made possible because of the support and understanding of my wife, Cherna, without whom this book and my other books would not have been written.

INTRODUCTION

....

AFTER more than thirty years of working as a practicing gastroenterologist, I remain convinced that not only are gastrointestinal symptoms, such as heartburn, gas, bloating, and abdominal cramps very common, but also these symptoms can be so severe that they ruin the quality of life of many patients. Furthermore, I am convinced that most gastrointestinal conditions and symptoms have a physical basis that can be worsened by stress, anxiety, and the extremes of emotion. For the past several years I have been Chief of Digestive Diseases at UCLA, the world's largest division dedicated to the study and treatment of digestive diseases. Not a day has passed in which I have not seen or at least spoken to a number of patients with the common symptoms associated with irritable bowel syndrome, gastroesophageal reflux disease, abdominal pain, or a variety of related symptoms. I can easily sympathize with the perplexed patient who has had his or her life turned upside down by these conditions.

I began my career at the University of Chicago, where I attended medical school, and then I moved to the Johns Hopkins Hospital, where I served as an intern. At the

Mayo Clinic, I did my Medicine and Gastroenterology residency and also spent several years at the National Institutes of Health. I have been at UCLA since 1969 and have steadily moved up the ladder to my current position as Chief of Digestive Diseases. During the course of over three decades, I have produced more than 300 publications and been the author or editor of 63 books on digestive diseases. In addition, I have written chapters in 24 other books. I have been fortunate in being able to learn a great deal from my teachers as well as from my colleagues, my students, and especially from my patients. Much of what you will read in this book is derived from my experiences with these important people in my life. My approach to the management of gastrointestinal symptoms reflects more the art than the science of digestive diseases, for scientific investigation has not been adequately applied to our understanding of many of the most common symptoms and conditions. Thus, my approach may differ from that of other physicians; it reflects what I have found helpful to people in my practice. I am hoping that, over the coming years, proper clinical investigation will show us how to better manage these conditions.

FREEDOM

from

DIGESTIVE DISTRESS

1

Why Me? What Really Causes Heartburn, Gas, Bloating, and Irritable Bowel Syndrome— It's Not Just the Foods You Eat

···

FOR decades, some of the funniest and most memorable commercials on television have flooded our living rooms with images of uncomfortable-looking people suffering from acid indigestion, heartburn, gas, bloating, diarrhea, and constipation. Catchy tunes like "Pop, pop, fizz, fizz. Oh, what a relief it is!" encouraged us to take drugstore remedies, some of which come in rolls like candy, to "feel better fast." We laughed at pictures of oversized bellies ("What shape is *your* stomach in?") and overindulging consumers who groaned, "I can't believe I ate the whole thing!" And, today, as a host of newer (prescription and nonprescription) drugs promise us relief, we continue to swallow two big notions that drug advertisers want us to digest: (1) minor digestive disorders automatically warrant taking medicines, and (2) uncomfortable symptoms are an expected part of "living the good life" in our hectic society.

Check your medicine cabinet, briefcase, purse, glove compartment, or pocket. How many of these prescription

and nonprescription remedies do you own? When heartburn strikes, is your first impulse to pop a pill or chew a
mint instead of thinking about what brought the episode
on? How much money are you spending on medicine?
How much time has your physician spent teaching you
that you may not need to take any medication at all?

I've written this book to show you that common digestive symptoms, such as heartburn (acid indigestion), gas,
bloating, diarrhea, constipation, and abdominal pain
(stomachaches) can often be relieved through lifestyle
changes—and may not require medicines at all. Over the
past thirty years, hundreds of patients have come to me
with these symptoms, and, time and again, I have seen that
people often prefer or expect a prescription for medicine
instead of a recommendation that they change their
lifestyle. That's because they want a "quick fix" rather than
undergo the lengthy and sometimes difficult process of
permanently modifying diet, exercise, and other lifestyle
habits they are comfortable with. So one of the first things
I have to help them change is their attitude about health.

Are Digestive Disorders a Necessary Consequence of Today's Life?

Far too many people accept heartburn, gas, bloating, diarrhea, constipation, and abdominal pain as normal. They
chew rolls of mint-flavored antacid tablets, drink thick chalky
elixirs to coat their stomachs, or pop the latest indigestion-
relieving wonder drugs as appetizers before downing heavy,
spicy, or fattening meals and still consider themselves in relatively good health. I'd like to argue that they are mistaken.

Gastrointestinal health—and indeed, one's overall health—is influenced by the dynamic, ever-changing interplay of numerous physical, nutritional, psychological, and social factors. These include eating patterns we learned in childhood, or attitudes about food, dining patterns, food choices, stress and anxiety levels, our workplace environments, and the priority we give to regular exercise in our lives.

In this chapter, we'll take a look at the symptoms and causes of some of the most common types of gastrointestinal disorders, including irritable bowel syndrome (IBS) and gastroesophageal reflux disease (GERD) that consistently send millions of Americans to the doctor and drugstore. (Note: Gastroesophageal reflux disease is often just referred to as heartburn, because heartburn is the disease's most common symptom. Sometimes the condition is also called "acid indigestion.")

A staggering number of Americans—sixty to seventy million, or one in four—are affected by gastrointestinal diseases. In fact, heartburn, gas, bloating, diarrhea, and constipation are the most common causes for visits to primary care physicians. I'll explain how each of these digestive tract conditions can be influenced by physical, nutritional, psychological, and social factors, and in the following chapters I'll provide practical tips for combating them.

Factors That Can Affect Your Digestive Tract

Physical Factors

Certain physical characteristics of people who suffer from common GI disorders can affect the disease. For instance, in a person with irritable bowel syndrome, the lining of the intestine is extrasensitive to a variety of stimuli, more so than in other people. So, for example, when the person's abdomen becomes distended (swollen) from eating gas-producing foods like cabbage and broccoli, it may cause tremendous pain and discomfort, whereas in a person who does not have the sensitivity, the same amount of distention will not cause any significant pain or discomfort.

Another physical factor that causes a digestive condition is infection with a bacteria called *H. pylori,* which causes some people to suffer from peptic ulcers. Still another is a weakened muscle called the lower esophageal sphincter (or LES), located between the stomach and the esophagus—the food pipe. This weakened muscle allows stomach acid to back up toward the throat, causing heartburn or acid indigestion. Even gravity contributes to heartburn in many people who lie down or recline too soon after eating a large meal.

The Effects of Smoking

Smoking produces both overt and hidden deleterious effects on the gastrointestinal tract. When you inhale smoke, a lot of it gets into your gastrointestinal tract. This will manifest itself as a sensation of gassiness, bloating, rumbling, gurgling, and even cramping. More importantly, smoking can be associated with serious injury to the gastrointestinal tract. For example, nicotine stimulates acid production, therefore, it promotes acid reflux, as well as worsening peptic ulcer disease. Smoking is clearly associated with an increased risk of cancer of the esophagus and cancer of the stomach. The mechanism by which smoking

invites the development of cancer isn't completely understood, but the association remains strong.

A fifty-two-year-old businessman came into my office
with a long list of gastrointestinal complaints, including
belching, bloating, rumbling and gurgling, abdominal
cramping, and recently difficulty swallowing. He'd had
these symptoms for years, but he was always "too busy" to
do anything about them. Accordingly, he had never taken
any acid-reducing drugs, made any lifestyle changes, or
even been evaluated. His symptoms were characteristic of
irritable bowel syndrome, which had been aggravated by
the ingestion of smoke over the years. His smoking two to
three packs per day was clearly worsening his underlying
condition. However, his trouble swallowing suggested that
he had developed either an inflammatory stricture in the
esophagus or esophageal cancer. Accordingly, he underwent upper endoscopy and our worst concerns were realized. He, indeed, had cancer of the lower third of the
esophagus. He underwent extensive surgery, but survived
only nine months. He was a victim of his lifestyle.

Nutritional Factors
Certain food choices can trigger or worsen gastrointestinal
disorders. Obviously, poor dietary choices can lead to
excess weight gain, which in turn causes a multitude of
health problems. It's amazing to note that we are seeing an
increase in dietary-related medical conditions as our society becomes more affluent. Even though there are more
wholesome foods available today than perhaps ever before,
we are making poor food choices. For example, while our
grandparents ate a relatively well-balanced diet of grains

and vegetables with little meat and occasional sweets, today's average American diet is far too high in fats, protein, sugar, and salt—and it's short-changed on complex carbohydrates. One reason for this epidemic of poor eating habits may be the availability of fast-food restaurants that offer taste-tempting, filling foods—like hamburgers, fried chicken, and burritos—for moderate prices. Many people who are working longer hours find it advantageous to stop at these fast-food restaurants or delis and pick up fat-laden, ready-to-eat dinners on their way home from work.

For many people with digestive disorders, the most obvious but least-followed nonmedical therapy is following a proper diet. However, reworking a diet to alleviate or eliminate a GI condition requires more than the elimination of junk food. Even healthy foods can aggravate the systems of those with heartburn, gas, bloating, constipation, diarrhea, or stomach pain. For example, cabbage, broccoli, and beans are healthful, nutritious foods for most people, but they cannot be tolerated by people who suffer from gas and bloating because these foods produce gas in the digestive tract. In the same way, milk and milk products are healthful sources of protein and calcium for most people, but they can aggravate gastrointestinal symptoms in those who are lactose-intolerant.

The problem is that there is no single diet that will work well for all people with digestive problems. I can't just hand my patients a preprinted list of foods to eat and foods to avoid. Because each individual is unique, we must examine what foods he or she has been eating and how those foods have affected his or her symptoms.

In chapter 3, I'll outline a game plan to get your diet back in proper balance and help you uncover which food choices are apt to wreak havoc on *your* particular digestive tract. I'll show you how to keep a journal and use it to determine which foods are causing your digestive symptoms. If you're like many of my patients, you'll be surprised to learn that some foods you thought were causing you trouble aren't really the culprits after all! Then, I'll show you how to use the information you gather from your food journal to help you create your own personal food guide pyramid—a personally customized version of the original USDA Food Guide Pyramid—that will help you eat a balanced diet and avoid your unique set of GI symptoms. I'll also give you tips for gradually starting to make changes to your diet in ways that will help you change your eating habits permanently—without being unhappy about it.

Psychological and Social Factors

In many people, especially those with irritable bowel syndrome, stress and anxiety can influence GI health as strongly as food choices. Your self-esteem and general outlook can also affect GI health. Further, our social lives are awash with alcohol and irregular dining habits, which spell bad news for GI health. In this book we'll dig deep into how social conditions influence behavior, which in turn can have a profoundly negative effect on the digestive system.

Over the past thirty years, I have observed broad changes in my patients' dietary and lifestyle habits. Nearly all of my married patients are part of dual-income families, in which both partners work to make ends meet. My patients generally work longer hours, bring work home, and take fewer vacations. Cellular phones keep them connected to the office day and night. To relax, they self-medicate with "comfort foods," alcohol, and the television remote control. Despite warnings posted on cigarette packs about the increased risk of health problems connected to smoking, many still light up. One of the most striking changes I have seen is how much less exercise my patients get today compared with a couple of generations ago. As machines and computers have made our daily lives easier, we humans no longer have to perform many physical tasks—like washing clothes with a scrub board or tilling the soil to grow food for dinner—chores that gave our ancestors a good workout. More and more of us have sedentary jobs. We ride to and from work in automobiles—parking as close to the building as possible—or take public transportation, take elevators instead of climbing stairs, and then sit most of the day engaging in little physical activity other than typing on a keyboard or lifting a telephone receiver. While we once got up from our chairs and walked down the hall to talk with coworkers, we now send e-mail messages. Thanks to modern conveniences, from garage-door openers to drive-through car washes to remote TV and stereo controls, physical activity has often all but disappeared from our daily lives.

Let's look at two of the most common digestive disorders that plague Americans today—irritable bowel syndrome (IBS) and heartburn (the primary symptom of gastroesophageal reflux disease, or GERD)—to see how these factors influence these problems.

Irritable Bowel Syndrome (IBS)

Michelle has irritable bowel syndrome. She'd had "stomachaches" throughout her childhood, and often these would keep her from attending school. Her parents took her to a pediatrician several times because of the pain in her abdomen, but her doctor never found a physical cause for it. After that, Michelle's parents began to wonder if she was just imagining her stomach pain—or perhaps making up the symptom to avoid classes. Sometimes, when Michelle asked to stay home from school because of her discomfort, her mother would say, "Now, Michelle, remember that the doctor said there's nothing wrong with you. Try not to think about it and it'll go away. It's all just in your head."

In her teenage years, Michelle developed abdominal gas and bloating. She was concerned and sometimes embarrassed by all the rumbling and gurgling that was going on in her abdomen. She also started having diarrhea that sometimes alternated with bouts of constipation. The diarrhea was particularly troublesome because it often arrived with a sense of urgency to find a bathroom—would she make it in time? Because of this she sometimes opted not to attend events like sports events or camping excursions with her schoolmates. When constipation was her problem, it caused her quite a bit of abdominal discomfort, so she preferred to stay home then, too.

As she entered her early twenties, Michelle had become a beautiful and talented artist who showed great promise in designing fashionable clothing, but she found her life revolving more and more around her gastrointestinal symptoms. She participated only in activities that took place in familiar surroundings—where she knew she could quickly find a bathroom. She passed up chances to go skiing or hiking with her girlfriends because she didn't want to get caught on a ski lift or mountainside when an attack of diarrhea struck. She avoided going out on dates because she didn't want her companions to discover her embarrassing symptoms. She feared they would hear her rumbling, gurgling stomach; she knew from years of experience that the stress of trying to make a good impression would only send her running to the bathroom. So she made up excuses and stayed home.

Michelle's irritable bowel syndrome affected far more than just her digestive tract. It affected her whole life. She was sad and lonely because of it, and felt that she couldn't discuss her symptoms with even her closest friends. Who would want to hear about her diarrhea? Besides, her mother had taught her that such subjects were not to be brought up in polite company. So she suffered in silence and spent evenings and weekends alone with her sketch pad. In an attempt to solve her problem, she saw many physicians and underwent repeated testing. Eventually, she was referred to me.

In her first visit to my office, Michelle had great difficulty in relating her story and avoided revealing the details about the nature and severity of her symptoms. In order to make it easier on her, I decided to go slow and take not one but several sessions to investigate her history and to get a better understanding of her condition. I also decided that it wasn't necessary to repeat her tests. They had been performed several times already, and everything seemed in order. Tests had ruled out cancer or any other serious illness, so I felt fairly sure that she had irritable bowel syndrome (IBS).

I explained to Michelle that irritable bowel syndrome is a common disorder of the intestines that affects roughly one out of five people in the United States, and often begins in adolescence. Three times as many women as men are affected. Symptoms of irritable bowel syndrome include abdominal pain, cramping, gassiness, a bloated feeling, nausea, loss of appetite, and changes in bowel habits. Symptoms vary from person to person. Some people have constipation (difficult or infrequent bowel movements); others have diarrhea (frequent loose stools, often with an urgent need to move the bowels). In others, constipation and diarrhea alternate, at times with drastic swings from one to the other. Sometimes the person with irritable bowel syndrome has a crampy urge to move the bowels but cannot do so. IBS can be merely an occasional nuisance or a mild annoyance, but it can also be disabling and cause sufferers to withdraw from normal activities. Feeling the need to be near a bathroom can prevent them from attending social events, going to work, or even leaving their homes. Irritable bowel syndrome is a problem that's inconvenient at best, incapacitating at worst, and almost always embarrassing to discuss with family and friends.

The cause of irritable bowel syndrome is unknown. Doctors call it a functional disorder because medical tests often reveal nothing to explain the symptoms and there is no sign of disease when the colon is examined. However, we do know that people who suffer from irritable bowel syndrome produce chemicals in the brain called neurohormones. In IBS patients, these chemicals adversely affect gut motility (the movement of material through the intestines). Further, their intestines tend to have a lining that is more sensitive to irritation—from the presence of certain foods in the intestine—or distention—swelling of the intestine in reaction to food—than people without this condition. Because of this extrasensitive intestinal lining, people with IBS experience pain that other people do not. Irritable bowel syndrome causes a great deal of discomfort and distress, but it does *not* cause permanent harm to the intestines and does *not* lead to intestinal bleeding or to a serious disease such as cancer.

Ordinary events such as eating and abdominal swelling from gas or other material in the colon can cause the colon to overreact in the person with irritable bowel syndrome. Certain medicines and foods may trigger spasms in some people. Sometimes the spasm delays the passage of stool, leading to constipation.

Researchers have found that women with irritable bowel syndrome may have more symptoms during their menstrual periods, suggesting that the reproductive hormones can increase irritable bowel syndrome symptoms.

When I told Michelle, "The good news about irritable bowel syndrome is that there are a lot of things you can do for yourself to help relieve the symptoms," she seemed pleased. Then I said, "First, I'd like you to start getting some physical exercise each and every day."

Michelle told me that she enjoyed swimming and she also liked going for walks. I encouraged her to do both, but that when she walked, she should walk briskly. I suggested that she should walk by herself so that she wouldn't get involved in conversation with her walking partner, which would only slow her down. She started with 15 minutes of exercise daily and gradually built up to 60 minutes per day. (I'll talk more about exercise in chapter 4.)

How Diet Can Affect Irritable Bowel Syndrome

I also explained to Michelle that what she ate could affect her condition, too. Many people with irritable bowel syndrome report that their symptoms occur shortly after a meal. This is because eating causes contractions of the colon. Normally, this response may prompt an urge to have a bowel movement within thirty to sixty minutes after a meal. In people with IBS, the urge may come sooner, along with cramps and diarrhea.

The strength of the response is often related to the number of calories and the amount of fat in the meal eaten. Many foods are high in fat, especially meats, poultry skin, whole milk, cream, cheese, butter, vegetable oil, margarine, shortening, avocados, and whipped toppings. Chocolate, milk products, beans and other gas-producing foods, or large amounts of alcohol are also frequent offenders. Caffeine causes loose stools in most people, but it is more likely to affect those with irritable bowel syndrome.

Excess fiber, in some cases, may make symptoms worse. Although fiber may be helpful in treating constipation, its use to relieve abdominal pain and diarrhea associated with irritable bowel syndrome is controversial.

I recommended that Michelle avoid uncooked fruits and vegetables (as in salads), but encouraged her to eat well-cooked fruits and vegetables for their fiber content. I also recommended that she drink fruit and vegetable juices for their vitamin content, and that she drink six to eight glasses of liquid every day. I asked her to take psyllium or a predigested vegetable powder—both are available in health food stores and most drugstores—each morning.

Living with Irritable Bowel Syndrome

Over a period of several weeks, Michelle's symptoms lessened in severity and frequency, and she began having more good days than bad days. But then she accepted a new job as a designer at a major clothing manufacturer, and she returned to my office once again complaining of diarrhea. "It happens every time I have to present my designs to the committee," she said. "I wake up the morning of the presentation with my stomach in knots and I just want to call in sick and stay home."

Stress stimulates colonic spasms in people with irritable bowel syndrome. While stress may worsen symptoms of irritable bowel syndrome, it's important to recognize that it is *not* a psychosomatic illness nor is it the result of a personality disorder. The symptoms aren't "all in your mind."

I pointed out to Michelle that nearly everyone has experienced the connection between the mind (emotions) and the gut at one time or another, whether it was a sensation of having "butterflies in the stomach" before delivering a speech or awakening with a "bellyache" the morning of an important exam. In IBS sufferers like Michelle, though, the link between the gut and emotions may simply be stronger than in most people. Stress and anxiety don't *cause* irritable bowel syndrome, but they can aggravate its symptoms. Many people can connect the onset of their symptoms to specific, often upsetting, events in their lives, while other people who suffer from irritable bowel syndrome find that it is brought on by routine, everyday stress.

I told Michelle that I didn't think staying home from work every time she felt stressed was a good strategy: "The goal is to help you find relief from your symptoms by increasing your ability to deal with—not avoid—the people and situations that cause them." Stress reduction can help relieve the symptoms of irritable bowel syndrome in some people, so I recommended that Michelle try practicing relaxation techniques. (I'll talk more about these in chapter 5.)

We then discussed other strategies she could use to try to reduce her stress. I asked her what was the worst thing that would happen if the design committee didn't like her sketches. "Would they ridicule you? Would your boss fire you?" Michelle smiled and admitted, "No, they'd probably just have me redo them for the next meeting." Using exercises like these, Michelle was able to begin to put her worries in proper perspective and limit her stress. I also recommended that Michelle go for a walk or swim on those mornings when she woke up stressed because of an upcoming presentation, because exercise is a wonderful stress reducer.

Many people with irritable bowel syndrome have benefited from meditation or relaxation techniques. Other techniques to reduce stress include getting regular physical exercise, improving communication skills, and practicing time and money management. (We'll discuss these strategies as well in chapter 5.)

Not every patient with irritable bowel syndrome is like Michelle. Let me tell you about Lenny, an aspiring actor who supplemented his income waiting tables. Lenny had a different set of symptoms than Michelle, so we came up with different ways to combat them. Lenny had suffered from a "nervous stomach" since he was a boy. He was his mother's favorite child, and she doted on him. He was a shy boy, and he disliked meeting new people, standing up in front of a group, or in any way calling attention to himself. His stomach tied up in knots whenever he had to perform in a piano recital or recite a poem in front of his class at school, even though he was a fair pianist and was quite good at memorizing and delivering poems.

Over the years, with his mother's help and encouragement, Lenny tried to overcome his fear of public speaking and performing. He took various music lessons, including voice, piano, and flute, and he learned to tap-dance. Each of these activities required him to perform in recitals from time to time. And each time he had to perform, his stomach would hurt and he would feel bloated. Sometimes he worried that he would belch or pass gas in the middle of a performance.

Interestingly, when he graduated from high school, despite his fear of performing before an audience, Lenny decided to pursue a career in the theatrical arts. He went to an arts college and found that he was able to manage his stomach pain, gas, and bloating by practicing his material so well that he was no longer nervous when he went onstage. But if he ever felt unprepared and thus stressed, the symptoms flared up.

Just prior to his coming to see me, Lenny had an opportunity to play a minor role in a television program. It was the break he had been waiting for. He practiced and practiced his lines, and he rehearsed with all his heart and soul. But then, on the first day of shooting the pilot episode, Lenny experienced a terrible attack of diarrhea. It was so bad he had to go home in the middle of the day's shoot. He was mortified. He didn't answer his phone when they called from the set to see if he was all right. The role went to someone else. Lenny felt this just might signal the end of his career.

But, after sulking for a few days, Lenny took his mother's advice and went to see his family doctor, who diagnosed his irritable bowel syndrome and referred Lenny to me for treatment. I liked the young man from the start, and enjoyed his quick wit as he told me the story of his horrible bout of diarrhea. Because his symptoms were so clearly triggered by stress, I told him we might first try to help him learn to manage his stress instead of treating his symptoms with medicine. Lenny agreed.

I asked Lenny to begin keeping a journal to record everything he ate; how he felt before, during, and after eating; who he ate with; and to list any symptoms he experienced. We examined his journal entries at his next visit, and we began to detect some patterns. For one thing, we found that Lenny had a habit of drinking several cups of black coffee and smoking many cigarettes while he was studying and rehearsing. He was always watching his weight, so he ate a lot of salads. I pointed out to him that both coffee and raw vegetables are common causes of diarrhea in people with sensitive digestive systems, and that raw vegetables cause gas in many people. Then I explained that Lenny's cigarettes were likely contributing to his gas and bloating. In the process of smoking a cigarette, you inhale and swallow air. Swallowed air is one of the major causes of gas, bloating, abdominal swelling, and belching. Lenny and I were gradually piecing together the puzzle of what factors were contributing to his symptoms.

Because stress clearly worsened Lenny's symptoms, we talked at length about how people react to it. I explained that, whether confronted with a frightening event such as seeing a car suddenly pull out in front of you when you're on the highway or an ongoing tension in your life, like dealing with a difficult boss, your body's physical response to the stressor is similar in each case. Your body gears up to "fight"—that is, face the challenge—or "take flight"—that is, muster the strength to move out of harm's way. In fact, your body reacts the same way whether the stress is physical or emotional, real or imagined.

I told Lenny that he might sometimes be contributing to his own stress by blowing situations out of proportion in his mind. Just as I had done with Michelle, I asked Lenny what was the worst thing that would happen if he forgot a line or misspoke. "They'd tar and feather me," he quickly answered in jest, showing that he knew he was exaggerating. Then Lenny told me about a trick an actor friend uses to overcome fear of making a mistake on a new job. "Geoffrey told me that he tries to hurry up and make that first mistake—he sometimes actually stumbles over a line on purpose—just to get it over with. With that, he proves to himself that nothing too horrible happens if he makes a mistake. The tension is eased so he can go on with less stress." While this tactic might not work for every actor, it serves as a stress-reducing strategy for Geoffrey—and now also for Lenny.

I also introduced Lenny to a meditative technique called the relaxation response (described in chapter 5) in which a repetitive word, phrase, sound, or movement is used to elicit a physical response that is the opposite of the response we feel to stress. When faced with a stressful situation, many of my patients find that this simple exercise can have an immediate calming effect.

One of the most important recommendations I made to Lenny was that he begin a program of regular physical exercise. Because he said he enjoyed dancing, I suggested he enroll in an aerobic dance class. He didn't like the first one he tried, but eventually he found one to his liking and began attending regularly on Monday, Wednesday, and Friday mornings. I think it's important for people to exercise each and every day, so I encouraged Lenny to try walking on the days when he didn't have class. Walking is often an especially effective stress-reducing exercise because the repetitive pounding of your feet on the pavement can elicit the relaxation response. The combination of stress-reduction techniques and exercise made quite a difference in how Lenny was feeling. His overall well-being improved and he has not experienced a recurrence of his diarrhea. By watching his diet, he is able to manage his gas and bloating. I hear that he's auditioning for a new part in a television sitcom, and I think he'll do just fine.

Patients are often their own best doctors. Many of them get to know their bodies and their needs and can sense when something is right or wrong. In the next example, you'll see how one of my patients used her food diary to understand her illness and then develop strategies, including the use of a personalized food guide pyramid to manage her symptoms without medicine.

A thirty-four-year-old woman named Alice came to me for a routine annual physical. In talking with her, I learned that she had experienced irritable bowel syndrome for many years, but that it was no longer a problem because she had learned to manage her symptoms fairly well. She had first started to develop stomachaches in her teenage years especially in periods of anxiety, such as during final examinations at college. Often these stomachaches were accompanied by diarrhea. Eventually, her symptoms included gas, bloating, abdominal cramps, and alternating constipation and diarrhea. She'd seen many doctors and received many different tests to try to diagnose her condition, and she had tried a variety of treatments with little success. On multiple occasions, she had abdominal X-rays, and she had undergone a series of tests—colonoscopy and barium X-ray of the upper gastrointestinal tract—on three separate occasions. A variety of blood studies were consistently normal. She had also seen a psychiatrist, with little benefit. She had seen several gastroenterologists—doctors who specialize in diseases of the digestive tract—but none seemed able to help her. All of them, however, agreed on the diagnosis of irritable bowel syndrome.

Alice then began to analyze her own symptoms, and found that her gas and bloating with abdominal cramps were most severe during periods in which she was trying to lose weight, when she would confine her diet to salads and raw fruits. She also found that she had more frequent bowel movements during these periods, but at other times, when she wasn't under stress, she frequently developed constipation. She observed that fiber seemed to help relieve her constipation, but it increased her diarrhea and would often bring on increased gas and cramps. She noted that cabbage, broccoli, and Brussels sprouts, even when well cooked, seemed to give her more gas. Finally, she observed that on days when she took aerobics class or went for a brisk walk, she seemed to have less gas, bloating, cramping—and more normal bowel habits.

A food diary helped her make these observations, and accordingly she placed herself on a diet that excluded raw fruits and raw vegetables, especially salads. She also avoided cooked broccoli and Brussels sprouts. She read that charcoal could help relieve gas, so she purchased charcoal tablets from a drugstore and took them after meals and at bedtime.

Whenever she was constipated, Alice would take additional fiber in the form of predigested vegetable powder that she purchased from a drugstore. She also did some form of aerobic exercise daily, alternating swimming with running. With this regimen, her symptoms improved dramatically. She'd helped herself by tuning in carefully to the foods that bothered her specifically, and figured out that exercise eased her symptoms. I couldn't have done a better detective job myself!

Heartburn and Gastroesophageal Reflux Disease (GERD)

Now let me tell you the story of Ryan, a patient who came to me experiencing heartburn. Ryan was an aggressive, hardworking account executive in an advertising firm. His job was secure only as long as the account he managed remained with the firm. In order to keep his client happy, Ryan found it necessary to work long hours; he had little time for exercise or relaxation. He would often skip meals throughout the day and have a large meal—usually Mexican or Italian take-out he picked up on his way home—at night. Ryan developed the habit of unwinding with a before-dinner martini and a couple of glasses of wine with his meal. Soon after dinner, he would go to bed, where he would read for an hour or so before falling asleep.

With this routine, Ryan started gaining weight at a rate of about ten pounds per year. He also began experiencing a vague indigestion that occurred off and on throughout the day and evening. He started carrying mints in his pocket—isn't that what everyone in the commercials does?—and often popped one in his mouth because he liked how the mint flavor got rid of the bitter taste that frequently was present in his mouth. He continued on like this for quite some time, still working long hours and eating a heavy meal right before retiring each night, and, despite his warning symptoms, considered himself a normal, healthy individual. Didn't everyone have indigestion now and then?

After five years of this lifestyle, he developed frequent heartburn, a burning sensation in the back of the throat, a bitter taste in his mouth when he got up in the morning and then off and on throughout the day, and sometimes a sensation of food coming up into his throat. Eventually he started having what his coworkers considered frequent "colds," in which his voice would become hoarse and he would cough a lot and sometimes lose his voice.

Ryan then started to wake up at night with heartburn

and, during the daytime, food would sometimes "stick" in the middle of his chest. That's when he decided to come to see me, as he said, "for some medicine to get rid of the symptoms."

Instead of just handing him a prescription for medicine, I thought it was important to spend some time educating him about the root causes of his condition. I explained to Ryan that heartburn—sometimes also called acid indigestion—is a symptom, not a disease. In the United States, more than one-third of all adults experience heartburn at least once a month. Heartburn is a burning sensation felt in the upper abdomen or behind the breastbone; it's usually accompanied by discomfort in the chest and a sour taste in the mouth. It's the result of gastric acid backing up from the stomach into the esophagus (the swallowing tube between the mouth and the stomach) and irritating its nerve endings. That sour taste is the taste of your stomach acid.

I showed Ryan pictures illustrating that the esophagus is a narrow, muscular tube that carries food from the mouth to the stomach. It's supposed to be a one-way route. The contents of the stomach are normally kept in the stomach by a band of muscle called the lower esophageal sphincter (or LES), at the bottom of the esophagus where it meets the stomach. The LES remains tightly closed except when you are swallowing food. When this muscle fails to close tightly, that's when you can get backing up, or "reflux," of stomach contents such as acid, food, or bile into the esophagus. Heartburn is the most common symptom of gastroesophageal reflux disease (GERD). Gastroesophageal reflux disease is a condition in which the LES muscle opens too easily and allows acid to splash into the esophagus, causing frequent episodes of heartburn. Even in healthy people, the LES may get forced open once in a while by an overfilled stomach—such as after Thanksgiving dinner—causing a bout of heartburn.

Many things cause the LES to open abnormally, such as being overweight, overeating, eating certain foods—such as citrus, peppermint, chocolate, fats, or spicy foods—caffeine, alcohol, and smoking. Pregnant women also frequently complain of heartburn, as the growing baby puts increasing upward pressure on the mother's stomach. Some weightlifters get heartburn because their activities produce pressure on the LES muscle. In addition, taking certain medications, such as aspirin and ibuprofen, can cause heartburn.

I asked Ryan if he were willing to undertake some reasonable lifestyle changes to alleviate his symptoms. When he said that he was willing, I gave him an overview of his options, the lifestyle changes that have worked for many of my patients:

- Lose weight if you are overweight.
- Eat moderate portions of food and smaller meals.
- Go for a walk after meals or at least remain upright. Reclining or lying flat (especially on your back) right after eating can produce intense acid reflux. Try not to eat meals in the three- to four-hour period before lying down.
- Cut out late-night eating. Avoid bedtime snacks.
- Raise the head of your bed by four to six inches to keep acid from backing up at night. This can be done

by putting blocks under the head of your bed or by using a special wedge-shaped support that elevates the top portion of your body. Extra pillows that raise only your head don't work—they actually *increase* the risk for reflux.

- Avoid bending over from your waist (especially after eating a heavy meal)
- Avoid wearing tight clothing and belts.
- Avoid alcohol, since it relaxes the lower esophageal sphincter (LES) and may also irritate the mucous membrane of the esophagus.
- Quit smoking. Smoking is a well-documented culprit that causes the symptoms of gastroesophageal reflux disease by relaxing the LES muscle. Smoking can also reduce overall LES muscle function and increase acid secretion. Stopping smoking has been shown to improve the symptoms of GERD.

TO CHEW OR NOT TO CHEW?

Chewing gum or even chewing on a toothpick thirty minutes after a meal has been found to help relieve heartburn in some patients, because chewing produces extra saliva, which neutralizes acid. However, chewing gum that contains oil of peppermint can relax the muscle between the stomach and the esophagus, leading to acid reflux. Chewing gum doesn't help all GI upsets, however. People who experience gas or bloating should avoid chewing gum because it can result in swallowed air, which adds to the amount of gas in the digestive tract.

Once I spelled out the overall plan, Ryan was ready to start. But I told him we weren't going to make all these changes overnight; instead, we would take them a step or two at a time. First I asked him to avoid large meals (especially at the end of the day) and not to recline for three hours after a meal. I recommended that he raise the headboard of his bed on four-inch blocks so that the head of his bed would be slightly elevated. I also advised him not to wear tight clothing (especially around his middle), noting that the clothes he was wearing that day were pretty snug. "It's hard to find anything in my closet that's not tight these days," he joked, referring to the fact that he'd put on quite a bit of weight.

Dietary Changes Can Combat Heartburn

In his next visit, I started talking with Ryan about his diet. Some dietary strategies to reduce reflux without taking medications include limiting consumption of fatty foods, chocolate, peppermint, coffee (even the decaffeinated kind), tea, cola, and alcohol. All of these things relax the lower esophageal sphincter (LES), allowing acid to back up into the esophagus and cause heartburn. Specifically, I told Ryan:

- Limit or avoid foods that can weaken LES tone, including garlic, onions, chocolate, fat, peppermint, spearmint, and coffee.
- Limit or avoid caffeinated drinks and decaffeinated coffee and tea, as these increase acid content in the stomach. Other acidic foods include citrus and tomato products.
- Limit or avoid carbonated beverages. These increase the risk for symptoms of GERD by bloating the

abdomen and causing pressure that forces acid to back up into the esophagus.

Because I knew it was essential for Ryan to lose weight to feel better, I advised him to begin lowering the fat and calories in his diet. We discussed several strategies for doing this, including keeping a food journal in which he wrote down all the foods he was eating each day. After reviewing his journal on his next appointment, I was able to recommend specific changes he could adopt, such as passing the Mexican drive-through restaurant on the way home and instead preparing a low-fat meal at home. He agreed to begin eating three ordinary-sized meals per day, instead of consuming his whole day's calories in the evening.

Over the next few months, Ryan learned to avoid irritating spices and eliminated alcohol. Next, he eliminated peppermint, chocolate, and fatty foods from his diet. As he began to lose weight and feel better, I advised him to add exercise to his regimen. Although he insisted that there was no time for exercise in his busy routine (I hear this from just about all my patients), I told him that was no excuse. We talked about ways that he could incorporate exercise into his schedule, including taking fitness breaks in the middle of the day, during which he could walk up and down the stairs or take a walk around the block. With a little creative planning, Ryan redefined his idea of what exercise could be and discovered that he actually could add exercise to his daily routine. And, after exercising for a couple of months, his weight dropped considerably and he found that he could once again fit into lots of the clothes in his closet!

As you can see, Ryan's lifestyle changes didn't take place overnight, and his symptoms didn't disappear overnight, either. It took time for him to adjust to his new habits, and it took time for the symptoms to improve. But eventually Ryan became a much healthier man—his sense of well-being improved and his heartburn disappeared.

Here's another way heartburn can affect someone. SueEllen was a forty-eight-year-old mystery writer who came to me complaining of an acidic taste in her mouth and a feeling that her food was sticking "like a big lump" in her chest instead of going down into her stomach. After performing tests ruling out serious inflammation of the esophagus, I concluded that SueEllen was experiencing acid reflux, a sign of gastroesophageal reflux disease. I told her that I didn't think she needed medicine for her condition, but that instead I'd like her to make some lifestyle changes. She told me that would be okay, "as long as it didn't take too long." She had a book manuscript due at her publisher's office in two weeks, and she hoped to be feeling well quickly in order to meet that deadline.

I explained to SueEllen that, while it would be nice, lifestyle changes don't happen overnight. Before we would even know what changes she needed to make, we would have to play detective and begin a very careful investigation of all the clues we could find. The mystery writer in SueEllen was intrigued by this discussion, so I added a bit of drama to my voice and said, "Any number of things could be causing your symptoms—perhaps the foods you eat, maybe the company you keep when you eat them, or maybe even your pants—if they're too tight around your middle. Like Sherlock Holmes, we will have to leave no stone unturned in our investigation." I saw the glimmer in SueEllen's eyes and I knew that she would enjoy this detective game.

I sent her home with the assignment to begin writing down everything about everything she ate in her food journal: the time of day, the place, what she ate, how she felt—both physically and emotionally—when she ate it, who was with her, and how she felt after eating. To make it more fun, I also asked her to write down anything *unusual* that she, as a good detective, thought she should note.

For her next appointment SueEllen arrived early, notebook in hand. We sat together and examined each entry, looking for clues. "I see a pattern here," she said. "When I drink coffee and smoke a couple of cigarettes in the morning after breakfast while I'm sitting at the computer, I get that lump in my chest. But when it's my day to stop at my daughter's house and give the grandkids breakfast and walk them to the school bus stop, I never seem to notice anything sticking in my chest."

I asked her what was different between the two situations. It turned out that when she was home by herself, she ate doughnuts and coffee for breakfast. But when she went to her daughter's house, she ate the same whole-grain cereal with fruit and low-fat milk she gave the kids. And, while she made a rule of never smoking around the grandchildren, she lit up frequently when she was writing at home. Using this deductive approach, SueEllen was able to see for herself that high-fat foods like doughnuts, as well as coffee and cigarettes seemed to contribute to her symptoms. I pointed out that the walk she took with the kids to the bus stop could be helping to combat her symptoms, too.

Over the following months, I guided SueEllen through the process of detecting foods and lifestyle habits that could be contributing to her particular GI symptoms. Then I instructed her to write a list of her findings. It looked like this:

- Avoid coffee: drink herbal tea instead.
- Quit smoking: go for a walk when you get the urge to light up.
- Avoid high-fat foods, including fried foods, butter, oils, mayonnaise, and cream. (These were the "comfort foods" SueEllen loved to make when she had writer's block.)
- Eat small meals, especially in the evening. (SueEllen often skipped meals if she was "in the writing groove" and rewarded herself with one giant blow-out of a meal when her workday was over.)
- Avoid eating within 3–4 hours before bedtime.
- Avoid wearing tight clothing, including "tummy control" underwear or pantyhose. (SueEllen liked to camouflage her weight gain with restricting undergarments.)
- Avoid bending over from the waist.

This was a good beginning. We then discussed other possible triggers for her symptoms and continued to outline ways to incorporate more GI-friendly lifestyle behaviors into her everyday habits. I feel that the more the individual patient participates in the process of uncovering his or her own personal symptom triggers, the more motivated he or she will be to make the appropriate lifestyle changes—permanently. Encouraging SueEllen to mentally walk through her day and discover the relationship between her food choices and symptoms was a revelation to her.

In the following chapters, I'll help you learn which lifestyle changes might help relieve *your* particular symptoms—and I'll provide you with lots of tips that I've gathered over the years from hundreds of my patients for ways to make these changes so that they'll stick for a lifetime.

2

The Insider Rules:
Ten Principles Guaranteed to
Get Your Gut Out of That Rut

....

T'S an undeniable truth: people tend to maintain the status quo, even if the status quo is ultimately harmful to
their health. Most people find it hard to make a
change—even if a favorite behavior causes pain or discomfort, like eating spicy food that tastes great but leaves you
with heartburn and an acid taste in the back of your
mouth.

People will go to amazing lengths to maintain equilib-
rium in their lives. They'll make countless little adjustments to try to avoid facing a potential health problem that
requires a major lifestyle change. For example, one of my
patients, a forty-nine-year-old aerospace engineer, was
referred to a cardiologist because his physician suspected
he had coronary artery blockage. When the physician
asked him if he had any discomfort that interfered with his
lifestyle, he kept saying no. In truth, he had stopped taking
the stairs at work because climbing stairs caused him to
have chest pains. So he had adjusted his habits just enough

to avoid having to tackle the problem head on. He risked his life rather than face the truth.

Because change is difficult for everyone, including people with GI problems, they often sidestep making needed lifestyle changes in an effort to maintain the status quo. I see people in my practice every day who are extraordinarily resourceful in avoiding major change. Some will buy clothes with elastic waistbands to avoid having to admit they've grown into a larger size and need to lose weight. Some people who have trouble sleeping at night because of acid reflux just stop going to bed at all—and begin spending their nights in recliner chairs watching old sitcom reruns and infomercials on television. To avoid uncomfortable symptoms, people will stop engaging in activities they used to enjoy—perhaps even stop having sex.

Many people try to self-treat their GI distress symptoms with over-the-counter medicines and ultimately fail because they're not addressing the root of the problem. For the great majority of GI sufferers, the key to successful symptom control is sticking to important healthful lifestyle changes—which, as we've discussed in chapter 1, can be done through an understanding of the interplay of the three key catalysts: the physical, the nutritional, and the psychological and social.

Over many years of watching people in my practice who avoid change, I've developed ten common-sense behavioral principles that can help people reclaim control over their digestive system—even if their lifestyle needs a complete overhaul. I call them *The Insider Rules*. I have found time and again that these core *Insider Rules* are a prescription for change, without medicine, that can improve the overall health and quality of your life—not just your gastrointestinal health. Note that some of the patient stories you'll read in this chapter are about people with serious GI diseases or conditions such as Crohn's disease or a duodenal ulcer. I include them to show extremes in behavior or lifestyle; even though your condition may be less "serious," you will learn much from their experiences.

1. It Takes More Than Resolve to Change a Habit

Crisis often precipitates changes, but those changes may prove short-lived. For example, most of us swear to stay out of the sun after suffering through a serious sunburn, but usually that resolve only lasts until the next sunny day. When a patient comes to me in anguish with symptoms of heartburn or irritable bowel syndrome, for example, I can bet that he or she will agree to go on a healthful, gut-friendly diet and exercise program—for a week or two. But once the crisis is over, old habits will creep back.

That's why it's not surprising that the same person who swears up and down, "I'll *never* eat spicy foods again!" when suffering from a painful attack of heartburn can turn around the following weekend and suggest, "Let's go Mexican!"

A patient who comes to mind has colitis due to Crohn's disease. He started smoking cigarettes when he was eleven years old. He is now thirty-nine and works as a carpenter and furniture designer. Nicotine clearly worsens the symptoms of Crohn's disease—a fact that had been repeatedly pointed out to this man by his family physician. Smoking caused him to experience severe abdominal pain, diarrhea, and cramping. Whenever he would have a particularly fierce attack of symptoms, his wife and three children would beg him to quit smoking. And he would kick the habit—just long enough for his diarrhea, cramping, and abdominal pain to go away. As soon as his symptoms were gone, he'd start smoking again.

As the years went by, his Crohn's disease worsened. He developed fistulas, which are spontaneous connections between loops of bowel or between loops of bowel and skin into which fecal material drains. He developed abscesses within the abdomen and signs of intestinal blockage, all of which led to a series of surgical procedures in which he had to have segments of his intestine removed. With each operation, he would quit smoking, resolving never to start again. But once the crisis was over, his nicotine habit would return. He recognized this pattern and joked that quitting smoking wasn't hard for him—"I've done it over a hundred times."

When he came in for a post-surgical checkup, I was finally able to discuss lifestyle changes with this man while he wasn't in the midst of a crisis. We calmly talked about various strategies he might use to quit smoking gradually, including using a nicotine patch to slowly break his physical addiction. He began right then to take positive steps to begin becoming a nonsmoker for good. When he came back to see me six months later, he was happy with his new nonsmoking life, and the symptoms of his Crohn's disease had eased considerably.

You need to resolve to make a change, but you also need to recommit yourself weekly, perhaps daily. From the outset, remind yourself that it's human nature to want to slack off when a problem eases—but that you're making a commitment to lifelong health, not short-term quick fixes.

2. Positive Reinforcements Work Better Than Fear

Fear can be a good motivator, but in the long run, it loses its charge. Showing smokers scary photographs of lungs blackened by a lifetime of smoking seldom has lasting impact on their decisions to light up. In a similar way, warning people with high-cholesterol levels about their increased risk of having heart attacks does little to change their behavior the next time they catch a tempting whiff of french fries as they drive by their local McDonald's.

Threatening remarks are especially likely to cause more harm than good when dealing with a person who has a digestive disease. The phrase "nervous stomach" is not just figurative. Anxiety has a decidedly negative impact on gastrointestinal health. I remember vividly a sixteen-year-old boy who was brought to me by his parents. Over several months, his pain had been increasing in severity and frequency, but he was afraid to tell his parents about it. Once I learned about his family situation, I understood why he chose to keep quiet about his symptoms. His parents had an unstable and unhappy marriage. His father, who consumed large quantities of alcohol and was often disoriented, had been an athlete earlier in life and had a long history of military service during which he received many promotions and honors, leading to his retirement as a major general. He and his wife taught their children that strength, success, and achievement were expected of them in all they did. Any kind of complaining was seen as a sign of weakness. Rather than complain about his abdominal pain and chance his father's calling him a "sissy," the boy chose to "tough it out."

The combination of the unhappy family situation, the demanding attitudes of his parents, and the young man's inability to achieve the levels of success in school and athletics his parents expected caused him a great deal of anxiety and fear. It wasn't until the boy's abdominal pain became unbearable and began radiating to his back that he finally had the courage to describe his discomfort to his mother. This led to the visit to my office. Long before he was brought to me for treatment, his pain had occurred infrequently—usually during periods of stress or anxiety or after he had eaten spicy foods. At that time, he found the pain could be temporarily relieved by drinking milk or eating. But now the pain was more severe and occurred more frequently.

After hearing the history of his symptoms and examining his abdomen, I was quite certain that, despite his young age, he probably had a peptic ulcer. In fact, an upper gastrointestinal endoscopy revealed the presence of a moderate-size duodenal ulcer.

I instructed the young man to avoid foods that caused his symptoms to get worse and to take some medicines—a proton pump inhibitor and two antibiotics that would kill the bacteria—called *H. pylori*—that causes duodenal ulcers. (We'll discuss these medications in chapter 6.) But I knew that medicine wasn't all he needed. We also had to deal with the anxiety and fear the boy was experiencing. Anxiety and tension increase the production of acid in the stomach, which, in turn, produces greater pain in a patient with an ulcer. I had a long discussion with the boy's parents and they agreed to curtail the anxiety-provoking remarks and threatening discussions that generated fear and anxiety in their son. I encouraged them to give their son positive reinforcement and praise instead of criticism. The parents cooperated and began to praise him for taking his medication, for continuing to attend school in spite of his discomfort, and for even minor scholastic achievements. The patient's response was remarkable—he not only rapidly became pain-free, but he also became a much happier, more cooperative, lively young man. This, in turn, led to a closeness within the family that had never previously existed. Within two weeks, his ulcer was healed. His teachers were pleased with the dramatic improvement in his attitude and in his scholastic achievements, and his parents marveled at the physical and emotional improvements that resulted from using positive reinforcement instead of instilling fear in their son.

In a similar way, when someone needs to change a lifestyle habit, such as exercising more regularly, threatening remarks are unlikely to scare them into action. Fright seldom inspires people to take positive steps for self-improvement. Plus, fear can sometimes cause another reaction—people become so afraid that they refuse to think about the subject altogether. That's why some people won't go for cancer checkups or cardiac stress tests—they're scared that they will find out bad news.

A seventy-six-year-old woman I've been treating for a few years comes to mind. Her husband died of colon cancer many years before I knew her and, unfortunately, her closest friend recently died of pancreatic cancer. My patient was in good health except for episodes of diverticulitis (an inflammation of the intestine), which responded well to conservative medical management, and irritable bowel syndrome with alternating diarrhea and constipation. Her symptoms were not severe and the cramping pain she sometimes experienced was easily controlled. At her annual physical examinations I recommended fecal occult blood testing (a stool test that detects traces of blood not visible to the eye) to screen for colon polyps or cancer. Because one of her parents had had colon cancer, I recommended that she have periodic colonoscopies (another type of test for colon cancer).

However, her fear of cancer was so overwhelming that she was virtually paralyzed in her thinking process about doing anything to screen for cancer in herself. She was fully cooperative during her annual physical evaluations and in the management of her IBS, but she refused any form of cancer examination screening. I made it a point to bring the need for it to her attention every six months, but she always found excuses to avoid such tests.

One day she came in complaining of fatigue and I evaluated her. For the first time I found that she was mildly anemic. Until then, she had always had normal blood counts, but now her hematocrit (a measure of the volume of red cells in the blood) was slightly below the normal range and her serum iron, which had previously been normal, was decidedly abnormal. I discussed all the possible causes for this change. Except for being tired, she was feeling perfectly well. With great reluctance and trepidation, she agreed to undergo a colonoscopy. She called me once or twice a day before the colonoscopy, expressing her fear and anxiety about preparing for the test and about taking the test itself. I assured her that the test was now done in such a way that people had no discomfort and, although the preparation required her taking an oral laxative, this, too, was not unpleasant.

Finally, the date of the colonoscopy came. She called wanting to cancel the test because she didn't feel up to it. I insisted that she come in and allow us to determine *why* she didn't feel up to it, and when she arrived, she agreed to undergo the test. During the colonoscopy, we found a large polyp on the right side of her colon that was bleeding. Within the polyp, there was a small mass of cancer. Fortunately, the polyp had not extended beyond the wall of her bowel or spread to other organs or lymph nodes. It was, in fact, curable. She underwent an operation to remove the cancer, and subsequently did well. But her fear of finding the worst almost resulted in a deadly situation.

It's important to build meaningful positive reinforcements into any program for behavioral change. If you lose ten pounds and everyone tells you how wonderful you look, that's often a good motivator to keep the weight off. However, not every change you need to make will have built-in positive reinforcement. Patients who need to reduce their cholesterol levels, for example, don't necessarily feel differently as their cholesterol levels drop. To provide a visual reminder of your success, you might want to post a chart on your refrigerator door or bathroom mirror. If your goal is to lose fifty pounds, for example, make a graph showing your weight at the end of each week. If you're trying to cut out caffeine or alcohol from your diet, put up a calendar and check off each day you successfully abstain from the item you're trying to avoid.

Make a list of the positive reinforcements you'll receive from changing your lifestyle, such as:

• I'll look better in my clothes.
• I'll feel more confident in public.
• I'll be ready to try more new things.
• I'll discover a new way of eating.
• I'll save money on cigarettes.
• I won't need caffeine to feel alert anymore.

3. Build In Appropriate Rewards

Changing your eating and other lifestyle habits takes work. People who suffer from digestive disorders often must give up foods they love. One way to encourage yourself to break bad food habits is to pat yourself on the back and reward your own good behavior.

In structuring rewards, ask yourself what you've been getting from the behavior you're trying to give up. For example, although smoking is a physical addiction, one of the rewards that often comes along with having a cigarette is companionship. Smokers associate smoking with sitting down with coworkers for a coffee break, or having a nice meal with friends. Smokers trying to kick the habit should make sure they give themselves the companionship associated with smoking without the smoking. A healthy alternative to asking someone to go for a smoke might be to invite them to go for a walk.

Be careful when planning rewards. In other words, if you're giving up cigarettes, don't substitute candy bars for smokes.

Too often, people reward themselves at the end of a long day at work with overeating, alcohol, or recreational drugs. These may provide escape routes from life's woes for a few fleeting minutes, but in the long run they cause more problems.

BEERS VS. BASKETS

One of my patients, a thirty-four-year-old advertising executive with heartburn who was trying to break the unhealthful habit of joining his buddies for a few beers after work, found that his friends were just as happy to go shoot baskets with him at the local YMCA. Because they were able to keep enjoying their after-work "unwinding" time together, the new habit stuck.

One of my patients, a thirty-five-year-old administrative assistant whose irritable bowel syndrome caused her to suffer from bouts of diarrhea alternating with constipation and bloating, started a walking program for exercise at my recommendation. She worked up to a thirty-minute walk each evening and was very proud of herself. I was surprised, though, that she wasn't losing any weight in the process. When I questioned her about her eating habits, she admitted that she had been walking to a neighborhood ice cream parlor and getting a double-scoop chocolate fudge cone each night to enjoy on the trip home as a reward for exercising. We discussed other, more healthy ways that she could reward herself, such as stopping by a local newsstand and picking up a favorite magazine, or relaxing in a hot bath when she got home. She started walking along another route, avoided the ice cream parlor, and soon began losing weight and feeling better. Six months later, she had lost ten pounds, and her diarrhea, constipation, and bloating had disappeared.

When planning healthful rewards for modifying inroads on changing your behavior, think back to your adolescence or childhood and recall activities you once enjoyed but haven't experienced in years. When was the last time you went bike riding, hiking, or ice skating? Allowing yourself time to experiment with a new hobby, such as oil painting, gardening, or woodworking can be a special treat. Activities that give you a chance to improve a skill seem to be especially rewarding. Working on your golf swing, learning to play the piano, or taking ballroom-dancing lessons can provide you with a healthful escape from life's routines and allow you to come away with a sense of accomplishment. An evening slumped in front of the TV with a bag of potato chips pales in comparison.

A forty-year-old laboratory technician who had experienced recurrent heartburn for many years came to me seeking relief. At the recommendation of his family physician, he had tried repeatedly to make changes in his lifestyle before, but he was always unsuccessful at sticking with the program. This time, he was ready to try to make the changes for life. I recommended that he help motivate himself by breaking the changes into small steps and rewarding himself for simple achievements. We drew up a plan whereby he would walk every evening when he got home from work—just a block or two at first, but gradually adding blocks until he was walking forty-five minutes daily. We discussed appropriate rewards for sticking with the walking program, and he decided that he'd really like to treat himself with something he'd always wanted to do but had felt was too extravagant.

REWARD YOURSELF

Think of rewards as anything you enjoy but don't get to do or to have often. Giving yourself permission to enjoy some leisure time can be one of the most important rewards for a job well done. An hour to read the newspaper in peace, a drive along the coast, a long bath, a chance to listen to some good music—anything that helps you get away from the toils of daily life. You're limited only by your imagination.

Here are some rewards my patients have used over the years:

- A day at a spa
- A massage
- A facial
- A pedicure or foot massage
- Tickets to a symphony or opera
- A day at the beach with a good book
- A ride in a blimp or hot-air balloon
- Tickets to the Super Bowl
- Lunch with your spouse—for no special reason—at a very special restaurant
- A relaxed visit to a bookstore to purchase audiotapes to listen to in the car
- A phone call to a friend from your past who now lives far away
- A *rare* food splurge, such as a hot fudge sundae, barbecued ribs, chocolate mousse cake, or baked Alaska (although I'd prefer that you indulge in angel food cake or other low-fat treats)

The reward he chose was to take up photography in a serious way. He had never before allowed himself the time to pursue this hobby because it required expensive equipment and would take up a lot of his time on weekends that he otherwise would have spent on do-it-yourself projects. When he had kept up his walking for two full weeks without fail, he took a trip to a local used-camera shop and bought some basic equipment. When he had logged another successful week, he permitted himself to sign up for a photography class at a nearby university. His walks soon became times for planning photo shoots and thinking about building a darkroom in his basement. His weekend getaways and vacations took on a new theme as he began selecting destinations that would make excellent picture-taking opportunities as well as good walking trails. The joy he found in his new hobby was the best stress relief he could have asked for.

FROM GOAL TO RESULT

When setting goals and breaking them down into specific manageable "bites," it's best to look for concrete behavior changes that you can make—and not confuse these "action steps" with the results you'd like to create. For example, if the *result* you want to achieve is to lose twenty pounds, your *goals* might be to eliminate alcohol (which contains a lot of empty calories) with your meals, to add a thirty-minute exercise workout to your daily routine, to cut down on added fats and oils in cooking, and to switch from doughnuts to low-fat cereal and skim milk for breakfast. Rather than rewarding yourself for losing a certain number of pounds, reward yourself for changing a behavior.

You may also be able to think of a hobby you've always wanted to try (writing a novel, learning to fly an airplane, or building a sailboat) that might serve as a good reward for you. Of course, the ultimate reward for making changes regarding your lifestyle habits will be how well you will feel when your symptoms of GI distress disappear!

4. Making a Change Requires a Positive Personal Plan for Action

Don't incorporate a punishing parent in your head. I recall three generations of a family I once treated. The grandparents, who came from a background of poverty, had worked long hours to provide basic resources for their two children. The husband was a salesman, whose job often kept him away from home, even on weekends and evenings. His relationship with his wife and children was loving but abusive. The children were expected to study each evening, finish their meals, observe a strict curfew, and show great respect for their elders. The father would respond to even minor infractions with verbal abuse *("You're no good!" "Can't you do anything right?")* and sometimes physical punishment.

The mother, a housewife, developed irritable bowel syndrome, with alternating constipation, diarrhea, cramping, bloating, excessive gas, and a feeling of incomplete bowel emptying when she went to the bathroom. Attacks of these symptoms correlated closely with confrontations between her husband and children. One of the sons developed recurrent stomachaches when he was twelve, and later developed alternating diarrhea and constipation, abdominal cramps, gas, bloating, and pain. These symptoms waxed and waned in severity, flaring up after periods of stress, anxiety, or confrontation.

The boy grew up, became a sales representative for a major food company, and married. His wife, like his mother, was condescending and quiet. He was authoritarian and abusive, both verbally and physically. They had one son, who eventually began complaining of abdominal cramping, pain, bloating, and diarrhea alternating with constipation. As this son grew into adulthood, I was able to help him understand that he was using "negative personal messages"—a habit of scolding yourself, instead of building yourself up ("positive personal messages"). I suggested that he may have learned this negative habit from his father—that was associated with worsening of his symptoms. Eventually, eliminating this negative self-talk, along with lifestyle changes including the development of a daily aerobic exercise program, a diet free of gassy foods, the use of charcoal tablets to relieve gas, and the occasional use of antispasmodic medications, he was able to take control of his life and his illness.

From a psychological standpoint, the language that we usually use in conjunction with life changes tends to have negative, authoritarian overtones. This language can often be traced back to childhood. Words like *discipline, control, willpower,* and *self-control* are often used to make children feel bad about themselves. I've found that many of my patients who have difficulty making changes designed to improve their gastrointestinal health had parents who were either authoritarian and controlling or, on the other hand, too lax in discipline. If you came from one of these kinds of backgrounds, you're likely to use negative phrases when talking to yourself, such as:

- I blew my diet again. Where's my self-control?
- I just don't have any willpower.
- I can't get myself to exercise.

ROOT FOR YOURSELF

Negative talk makes you feel bad and does nothing to help you change. Rather than punishing yourself with negative voices from the past, help yourself succeed. Remember, you're on *your* side! Instead of struggling against yourself, work *with* yourself to create a concrete plan of action that you can manage—and pat yourself on the back along the way.

If you slip off your new eating path, beating yourself up for transgressing will only make you feel like a child. It's better to assess the situation, analyze why you slipped, and then get back on the program. The same techniques work whether the lapse occurs when you're trying to start an exercise program or you're trying to stop drinking coffee. Review the reasons why the program will be beneficial, make specific plans for incorporating it into your schedule, and stick to those plans. Say these things to yourself:

- I don't have to be perfect.
- I can make small changes.
- Good for me! (on reaching milestones)
- Change is difficult for everyone.
- I can make the changes I want to make.

Making lasting change for digestive health is actually about increasing self-esteem and your ability to tolerate anxiety. By using the tools I'm providing you in this book—and by reinforcing your positive behavior with appropriate rewards as you go along—you can make lasting changes in your lifestyle habits.

Anything that builds your self-esteem and makes you feel good about yourself helps you work through the anxiety that's inevitable when the status quo gets shaken up.

I remember a twenty-two-year-old college student who complained of severe headaches and recurrent stomachaches. We subjected her to an extensive neurological evaluation and a complete gastrointestinal evaluation. No physical explanation for her headaches or her stomachaches was found. She was diagnosed with irritable bowel syndrome, even though she had not progressed to the point of having diarrhea, constipation, or cramps, but simply complained of recurrent aches in the pit of her stomach. After several visits, I grew to know her better, and it was clear to me that her self-image was poor. Both of her parents were highly critical of her activities. She had rarely received praise during her childhood or in her adult life. She felt insecure and inferior and generally felt unable to cope with what life dished out to her.

I recommended that she try to find an area in which she might develop skill, as well as get some joy out of life. I suggested that she try taking karate classes, because she was thin and agile, and I thought the structured format of karate might enable her to develop attainable goals. Reluctantly, she agreed to give it a try. Karate turned out to be "just what the doctor ordered." She caught on to the moves quickly and enjoyed working hard, knowing that she was improving all the time. Eventually, she achieved great prowess and recognition in the karate world. Her self-image dramatically improved, and for the past four years she has been free of headaches and stomachaches.

Even after you've quieted the negative voices in your head, you'll need more than willpower to achieve your goal. You have to make a real plan, with concrete steps to get you there one day at a time. This book will help you create that plan.

- *VISUALIZE SUCCESS*
- Picture yourself succeeding. If you're trying to quit smoking,
- picture yourself living smoke-free. If your goal is to lose
- weight, picture yourself wearing a favorite outfit you've out-
- grown.

5. Know Yourself: Understanding Your Likes and Dislikes Can Help You Tailor a Program That You Can Live with Long-Term

When you create an action plan, make sure it fits your preferences. For example, a noon fitness class might relieve tension and be a good source of exercise for some people, but might prove too stressful for you if you dislike group activities or hate wearing shorts. We are all different. We have different sensitivities, likes, and dislikes, too. This is true not only when it comes to how we live our daily lives but also with regard to what we eat and what we find relaxing. Above all, common sense is usually the wisest rule.

It's easy for me to make recommendations on diet and exercise, but I may not know the intricacies of your personal likes and dislikes. That's where you have to tailor the program to fit your needs. For instance, when it comes to exercise for the purposes of digestive health, vigorous exercise is really not necessary. For some people, vigorous exercise may be more enjoyable, but in fact a brisk walk will accomplish all of the goals listed in this book, as will a relaxing swim. Building up a sweat and raising the pulse may be helpful in cardiovascular health, but exercise in moderation generally is adequate for improving digestive health. If I draw up a healthful diet plan for you, it probably won't include your favorite healthful foods. (I've recommended some helpful resources for healthy eating in the Resources section.) Plus, if you design your own eating plan, you'll have more "ownership" of it and be more motivated to follow it.

- **LOOK TO THE PAST**
- Review your past accomplishments. What worked for you in
- the past is likely to work for you again. If you used to go to
- the gym more regularly when accompanied by a friend, then
- find an exercise partner. If, however, you know from experi-
- ence that you always stop going to fitness centers after the
- first month of your membership, then try another type of
- exercise—such as walking, dancing, or swimming laps.

Losing weight is often helpful in reducing gastrointestinal symptoms in obese patients. (Obesity is defined as being more than 20 percent over the recommended weight for your height.) However, weight loss is one of the most difficult goals to attain. Because many overweight people have had a lifelong battle with weight control, I find it useful to tap into their memories for strategies that worked for them in the past. I remember a patient with severe GERD who had such extensive reflux that acid was being aspirated into her lungs, causing chronic bronchitis, which made her cough frequently and lose her voice.

As she grew older, her heartburn grew somewhat better, but she developed a raspy voice and was constantly coughing. In spite of taking a variety of drugs, her cough and laryngitis wouldn't go away. These symptoms interfered with her daily life—she had trouble talking on the phone, she was shunned by others who didn't want to catch her ever-present "cold," and she was embarrassed by her harsh, grating voice.

It was clear to me that the more weight she gained, the more acid reflux she experienced. Not only did her weight influence the free passage of acid from her stomach into her swallowing tube (especially while she slept at night), but the large meals she ate invited reflux by their sheer volume. Plus, she made the situation worse by her habit of reclining soon after eating.

Overall, her quality of life was poor simply because she had lost control of her eating habits. Weight control had been a problem for her throughout her life—even before she developed digestive problems. Earlier in my care of her, she successfully lost fifty pounds by using a three-pronged dietary approach I recommended. First, I suggested that she eat all the foods she would normally eat, but cut her portions in half. This tactic gave her the satisfaction of tasting all the different foods she wanted, yet it reduced her total calorie consumption. However, she also needed to feel "full." To accomplish this, the second step was that she take a psyllium fiber supplement (such as Metamucil) before her meals. She had been taking a fiber supplement for many years to control her constipation, but she had been taking it at other times in the day instead of before her meals. Taking the fiber supplement *before* her meals would help fill her stomach and allow her to feel satisfied with a smaller amount of food. The third strategy we used was to increase her physical activity to reduce her stress-related hunger. I encouraged her to go for a pleasant brisk walk at least once every day.

Since this trilogy of strategies had worked for her earlier in life, I suggested she try it again. History repeated itself, and she did lose fifty pounds over subsequent months. Her self-image and general sense of well-being improved. She no longer suffers from heartburn, cough, or laryngitis. And, because she is also taking a fiber supplement, her bowel habits have returned to normal.

Many gastrointestinal complaints, especially those associated with irritable bowel syndrome and chronic dyspepsia, cause patients to become so frustrated that they're willing to try unproven treatments that seem to be helping other people. Sometimes this can get them into trouble. I remember one patient who suffered from irritable bowel syndrome for more than twenty years who did this. Even though she was getting plenty of aerobic exercise and had modified her diet somewhat, her symptoms continued. In an overzealous effort to nail down the dietary triggers that were causing her continued discomfort, she began eliminating many foods from her diet. If she ate some chocolate cake and experienced gas, bloating, and cramps afterward, she invariably blamed her symptoms on the cake—even though on several other occasions she had eaten cake without it causing symptoms. Eventually, she limited herself to a very restricted diet and slowly but progressively lost weight. What she didn't realize was that her symptoms were more severe during periods of anxiety, depression, and family confrontations. She also got advice from a number of friends and acquaintances, none of whom had exactly the same combination of symptoms that she experienced, but each of whom had certain digestive complaints, such as chronic constipation or diarrhea or excessive gas and bloating or abdominal swelling and discomfort. One such friend told her about the "miraculous" results she had experienced by taking a Chinese herbal medicine that was recommended to her by an herbalist who had a "fantastic" personality.

The patient was so frustrated with her symptoms that she was willing to try any kind of treatment that might bring her relief. She visited the charismatic herbalist and started taking herbs that he gave her in unlabeled packages. There was no way to know precisely what ingredients the packages contained. Three weeks later, she noticed her urine was dark and her husband noticed that her eyes were yellow. Her friends commented that her skin was yellow, too. She felt extremely tired, so she called me. I examined her and it was clear that she had developed liver disease. The results of her liver tests confirmed my suspicion—she had liver failure. She was hospitalized and eventually required a liver transplantation. She survived the difficult operation and has done generally well, but now she will have to take immunosuppressive drugs and have frequent checkups for the rest of her life. Her irritable bowel syndrome is no better or no worse, but it is clear her willingness to try an unproven treatment almost killed her.

- *NO TWO PATIENTS ARE ALIKE*
- Avoid comparing yourself to others. If you're walking, don't
- feel that you should be running just because joggers are passing by. Everyone progresses at his or her own pace. If you're
- doing better this month than you were doing last month,
- you're doing great.

    Avoid comparing your GI symptoms with those of others. Many of my patients who suffer from irritable bowel syndrome have compared their diarrhea or constipation, gas, or bloating to that of someone else and then tried a fad diet or unproven treatment—such as an herbal laxative—that worked for the other person. In general, this is a bad idea because no two patients are alike. What works for someone else won't necessarily work for you—and it may actually be harmful for you or make your symptoms worse.

6. Tackle Just One Major Change at a Time and Break Up Major Changes into Doable Steps

Trying to change everything at once is a guarantee of failure. I had one patient who was fifty-two years old and suffered from nearly daily episodes of severe heartburn. He also sometimes experienced pain in the middle of his chest when he swallowed and a bitter taste in his mouth when he got up in the morning. Often during the day a burning fluid would fill his mouth. He had smoked three packs of cigarettes a day for almost thirty years and was used to drinking one or two six-packs of beer each weekend, a couple of mixed drinks each evening when he got home from work, and wine with his meals. He was forty pounds overweight and frequently snacked on peppermints and chocolates. His family physician had diagnosed his condition as gastroesophageal reflux disease (GERD) and had recommended that he stop smoking, eliminate alcohol from his diet, avoid fattening and spicy foods, peppermint, and chocolate, and avoid reclining for at least three hours after eating. With great difficulty, the man instituted *all* of these changes at once.

After five days on this new regimen, his symptoms had improved greatly, but he felt nervous and unhappy. He felt as if he'd cut all the fun out of his life, and hadn't planned anything to take its place. He experienced an uncontrollable urge to return to the lifestyle he was used to. Within a week, he had abandoned all of the changes and returned to his status quo—and his heartburn, which returned worse than ever. If he had made these changes in his lifestyle one step at a time, it's much more likely that he would have been able to maintain them.

Many of my patients have found it works best for them to make the easier changes first so they have a foundation for success and increased confidence to make the harder changes. Once you've successfully incorporated a daily walk into your routine, for example, you'll be encouraged to try making another change, such as packing a healthful lunch for yourself when you get home from your morning walk. Then, once you've become accustomed to noshing on those healthful lunches, you may be inspired to take a stress-reducing yoga class after work. Over a period of time, your more healthful lifestyle will unfold—one change at a time.

Everyone approaches lifestyle and dietary changes differently. However, over the course of my career, I have found that for most people trying to eliminate a behavior, such as smoking or drinking alcohol or coffee, slowing to a halt is usually more successful than going cold turkey. It's much easier to take a series of small steps than to make giant leaps. Plus, small steps are key to effecting permanent change.

TAKE IT SLOW

To be most effective, any changes you adopt should be gradual. Gradual changes are less disruptive, and there's a better chance that they'll become an integral part of your life.

For most people, it's unrealistic to go on a diet expecting to eliminate all undesirable foods at once. If you suddenly deprive yourself of the foods you love and are accustomed to eating, you'll feel discouraged and are more likely to "cheat." It's better to gradually eat less of them. You're more likely to stick with changes if you tackle them a few at a time. Focus on making one or two changes until they become a habit. Then pick one or two new things to change. This way, you slowly change your eating habits. For example, fats in the diet are a major offender in exacerbating many GI distress symptoms. When you cut fats too drastically, your tastebuds don't have time to adjust to the new flavors and textures that come with low-fat eating. You also need time to practice new skills, such as ordering a GI-friendly meal at a restaurant or learning low-fat ways to cook.

So, the key to adopting a more healthful lifestyle is to do so slowly but surely. That way, the changes you're making won't fade after just a few weeks—instead, they'll last a lifetime.

Start making gradual changes in your diet today. But do only what you're ready to do. Find a habit or a food choice that you're willing to change right now. Once you've successfully incorporated more cooked vegetables and grains into your diet, for example, you might be encouraged to try making another change, such as substituting 2% milk for whole milk. After a week or two, switch to 1% milk, then gradually to nonfat (skim) milk. You might pick the area that needs the most improvement or you may decide to tackle the area that would be easiest to make changes in. You'll discover that many skills you use to make the easy changes will help you succeed in making more challenging changes later. Over time, you'll be eating foods that are more gut-friendly—without a great disruption in your daily life. It will simply feel natural.

In the same way, if you're trying to eliminate caffeine in your diet, start by cutting back on one cup of coffee each week. (If you quit coffee cold turkey, you could experience withdrawal headaches and lethargy, which could send you right back to the coffeepot.) Or if your goal is to walk three miles a day, you may need to start with just once around the block. Most of us have had the experience of charging into a new exercise program so enthusiastically that the next day's inevitable aches and pains benched us for a week. If you start more slowly, you'll be able to stick with it. As you gradually make these changes, congratulate yourself for making progress. Build in milestones that correspond to incremental accomplishments and celebrate without compromising all the good work done to date.

- ***IMPORTANT LITTLE STEPS***
- One of my patients reported that he could tolerate one small
- change every few days. On Monday, instead of ordering his
- usual tuna fish salad sandwich on a croissant, he ordered it
- on whole wheat bread. On Thursday, he felt ready to tackle
- another change, and he switched from the tuna salad with
- mayonnaise to sliced turkey with a little mayonnaise, again
- on whole wheat bread. A week later, he ordered the turkey
- sandwich with mustard instead of mayonnaise. Step by step,
- he was able to cut the fat from his lunches without too much
- disruption in his life.

7. Expect to Slip from Time to Time

If you're trying to lose weight and cut down on fats and chocolate, but you had two helpings of Aunt Patsy's chocolate cheesecake at your brother's fortieth birthday party, don't be dismayed. Changing your eating habits is sometimes a "two steps forward, one step backward" process. It's natural and expected that people will slip occasionally. Just know up front that holidays, special occasions, life's disappointments, and illness can distract you from your dietary-change goals. That's okay. Lapses will happen, so don't punish yourself or give up the program in the event of a minor slipup. Instead of hauling yourself over the coals after a lapse, try to figure out what triggered the slip. Then plan ways to avoid that trigger. Try to anticipate those situations that can trip you up. Sometimes planning ahead is all you need to do to prevent lapses. For example, special occasions don't have to be a problem. You can enjoy your food and companionship and still be good to your stomach. We'll talk more about making healthy food choices at parties and restaurants in chapter 3.

Another tactic I devised for one of my patients to help herself out was to remove obvious temptations. She was a forty-five-year-old secretary who had been diagnosed with severe heartburn, a symptom of GERD. She told me that she kept slipping with certain favorite food items, which for her were chocolate mint cookies, coffee fudge and mint chocolate chip ice cream, and chocolate-covered mint candies. I suggested that she remove these foods from the house, her desk drawer at work, or wherever else she might have them. At first, she insisted that she couldn't deprive the rest of the family of these treats, but she finally agreed that the others could get these unhealthy foods outside the home if they wanted them. Once these foods were out of sight, she was less likely to crave them. If she suddenly decided that mint chocolate chip ice cream sounded good at ten o'clock at night, she was much less likely to give in to that urge because she'd have to get dressed and go out and buy it. By ridding her environment of ready supplies of the foods she was trying to avoid, she suffered far fewer lapses.

When you do slip up, it's important to get back on the straight and narrow as soon as possible. Just because you eat a forbidden food at lunchtime doesn't mean the whole day (or weekend!) is a loss. Too often, people use a small slipup as an excuse to gut their plans to eat right and say, "I've already blown my diet for today—I'll start again first thing Monday morning."

Look for patterns in your behavior. Do you always abandon your healthy habits when you travel? This may be okay if you only travel on vacation once a year, but can be a serious problem if your business requires you to be a frequent flyer. Do you frequently overeat when you're lonely, bored, or sad, or do you always make poor food choices when you're with certain eating companions? We'll discuss ways to manage psychological and social triggers in chapter 5. Do you always skip your daily walk if the weather's not good? The solution may be as simple as creating an indoor backup plan for exercise on those days.

A forty-eight-year-old businessman who had experienced good health most of his life came to see me at the insistence of his wife and daughter because he'd been having recurrent episodes of heartburn. He described these attacks as intense burning sensations that started in the pit of his stomach and moved up into his chest, followed by a bitter liquid filling his mouth. When he woke up most mornings, he had a bitter taste in his mouth. On evenings when he had eaten large dinners, he would complain of severe heartburn and would self-medicate with whole rolls of antacid tablets. This was the first time in his life that he had ever had any significant illness. He was overweight and had gained almost thirty pounds within the past two years. He smoked cigars each evening, and also smoked at least a full pack of cigarettes each day. He was accustomed to having wine with his meals as well as one or two mixed drinks upon arriving home each evening. Three years ago, he'd given up his exercise program.

I advised him to undergo a gradual weight-reduction program and begin walking every day, slowly working up to forty minutes a day. I also recommended that he avoid wearing tight clothing, refrain from reclining for at least two hours after meals, and elevate the headboard of his bed. I told him to gradually start eliminating alcohol, caffeine, tobacco, and spicy foods from his diet. Within six months, he'd weaned himself away from cigarettes, alcohol, and coffee, and lost twenty-five pounds. He was walking almost an hour every day. And he was symptom-free.

Soon after I had seen him successfully managing his condition, however, stresses at his job became difficult for him to handle. He frequently worked late at night and delayed his dinner until nearly ten o'clock. He dropped out of his exercise program and regained much of his weight. In an attempt to relieve stress, he returned to alcohol and cigarettes, as well as to his habit of an evening cigar. Within eight weeks, his symptoms returned—and they were more severe than ever before.

Unfortunately, he had let minor slipups pile up until he had abandoned all the good habits he had worked so hard to cultivate. If he had found healthful ways to manage his stress, and stopped after each lapse and tried to figure out how to keep similar slipups from happening in the future, it's likely he would have been able to maintain his healthy habits.

THE UPSIDE OF SLIPUPS

When you slip off your intended program, consider it a learning experience. Try to figure out why the lapse happened and how you can avoid it next time.

8. Social Support Is Important

Get other people rooting for you. Enlist the support of your family and friends in your efforts to change your habits. For example, most meals are social events as well as opportunities to refuel your body. Even on occasions when your eating companions want to order a double-cheese pizza and beer, they may agree to have a veggie pizza with just a little cheese if they know you're trying hard to change your eating habits.

One of my patients who needed some major lifestyle overhauls was fortunate to have a very supportive family. His wife started cooking more healthful meals, and, when she explained to their teenagers how important it was that they encourage their dad's diet and exercise reforms, they decided that they could all do it together. They agreed to stop keeping potato chips, peanuts, and other junk foods in the house. The daughter asked her home economics teacher for some low-fat recipes. Every evening after dinner, his wife went with him for a vigorous walk. Whenever he said he didn't feel like walking, she'd coax him to go anyhow.

Working with my patients and their families, I've seen all too well the social politics of making a lifestyle change. Unfortunately, there's a possibility that some people will sabotage behavioral change in those they love. Remember, they want to maintain the status quo. They love you the way you are and they want you to stay that way. Plus, your lifestyle changes affect *their* status quo. If you commit to losing weight, your spouse may feel he or she needs to diet too rather than be the "heavy one" in the couple. If your family has developed a habit of celebrating Friday nights with a rented video and a bucket of fried chicken, your decision to make dietary changes and exercise more will impact their lifestyle as well. Remember, though, that your family members would benefit from a healthier lifestyle, and your good example may eventually rub off on them. The whole family might enjoy a softball game in the yard or a walk around the neighborhood after dinner.

- ***DON'T GO SOLO***
- If your family members aren't supportive of your efforts to
- make lifestyle changes, try to find support and encourage-
- ment elsewhere. It's harder to "go it alone."

It's easier to make and maintain changes when you're surrounded by people who support your efforts. So it's important to find a network of people who can be encouraging—outside support groups, exercise buddies, or a supportive spouse or friend can make the transition to a more healthful lifestyle easier and faster. With a little help from your friends, changing your way of eating can be more fun and more successful.

The thirty-two-year-old son of a famous self-made multimillionaire and politician came to see me because of irritable bowel syndrome that he'd had for more than twenty years. His illness was characterized by alternating diarrhea and constipation, abdominal swelling, gas, bloating, lower abdominal cramping, and prolonged periods of extreme tiredness. Throughout his life, he had a poor self-image. As a child, he had been thin and small, and failed to excel in any aspect of his life. He was a poor athlete and a below-average student. He was nearsighted and required thick glasses and his complexion had been marred by severe acne throughout his childhood and teenage years. As an adolescent, he had never had a lasting relationship, and in fact had rarely dated. Eventually, pressure from his parents forced him to attend college, where he did poorly academically, failed to be accepted by any fraternity, and had no real friends.

After college, his father had arranged a series of jobs for him, but none of them interested him. He failed to do well in any of these positions, but with the help of his family he managed to move from job to job. He consistently failed to achieve gratification from his work or in his personal life. During this time, his symptoms of irritable bowel syndrome progressively worsened and occurred more often, preventing him from participating in social or work-related activities.

However, an encounter with a woman at a coffeehouse changed his life. She was his age, and worked as a librarian. She led an active life that brought her great fulfillment. She was an enthusiastic volunteer for several charities and served as a mentor to two junior high school students. She was an avid reader of fiction and nonfiction, and shared her joy of literature by teaching after-school reading as a volunteer for a city-wide literacy program. She also loved to jog. In spite of the differences between the young man and this energetic young woman, their brief conversation at the coffeehouse led over a period of time to a close relationship. They dated regularly and her enthusiasm and love of life were infectious. She encouraged him to start exercising and he grew to love jogging daily through the city. He started slowly and eventually was running three to five miles per day. He lost weight, joined a gymnasium, and found great gratification in bodybuilding as he sculpted a torso he previously had not even dreamed of. As his social life improved and his physical appearance changed, he found that his stress and anxiety often were lessened by aerobic exercise. Gradually his abdominal symptoms virtually disappeared and his bowel habits became normal. Gas, bloating, and cramps were rare and became unimportant in his life. His quality of life greatly improved. He married the librarian in a quiet, private wedding ceremony. Although he remained distant from his family, he and his wife have developed a supportive and close relationship in which both of them have enhanced their self-image and achieved mutual understanding and self-esteem. He remains healthy and free of any physical complaints.

In some cases, I've seen patients whose family members or loved ones tried too hard to be supportive—and their constant nagging caused more stress for the person trying to change his or her lifestyle habits. One patient who had this problem was a sixty-seven-year-old retired businessman. His wife was always watching over his shoulder and reminding him that he shouldn't eat spicy foods, that he shouldn't have a drink in the evening, and that he shouldn't light up a cigar after dinner. He began to resent her reminders and referred to her as his "watchdog." Her watchfulness caused him to change his behavior, but not in the way we wanted it to change. Instead, he found lots of ways to "sneak" smokes, drinks, and favorite foods when his wife wasn't home or was busy talking on the phone or taking care of the grandkids. I talked with him about his behavior and we agreed that he wasn't taking responsibility for his own health. I suggested that he tell his wife that he'd like her to back off a little on the nagging and that he, in turn, would try harder to modify his habits.

9. Keep a Journal

One of the best ways to learn how what you eat affects the way you feel is by putting your food habits on paper. In order to make this exercise most useful, you'll want to write down not only what you eat but also what's happening to you and around you. By keeping a record of everything you eat, what time of day you ate it, and how you felt before, during, and after eating it, you can begin to get a clearer picture of your food and patterns. You'll begin to see which foods cause the most digestive problems and how healthful your overall diet really is. Do you eat a good variety and balance of foods? What proportions of your daily diet come from carbohydrates, proteins, fats, and empty-calorie foods (such as sugar and alcohol)? Do you grab junk food when you're in a hurry? How often do you eat fresh fruits and vegetables? How many cups of coffee do you drink? Many of my patients are surprised when they log their daily intake to learn how much fat they really are eating. Don't forget to include all the snacks you eat throughout the day—from the "samples" you nibble when preparing meals for the family to the spoonfuls of ice cream you sneak from the freezer in the middle of the night.

Your journal can help you separate *true* food-triggered events from happenstance. I clearly remember a sixty-three-year-old patient who had been suffering with chronic constipation, gas, bloating, and abdominal cramps throughout her adult life. She didn't keep a journal; instead, she trusted her memory. Whenever she would experience unpleasant digestive symptoms, she would recall what food she had eaten recently and would then eliminate that food from her diet—even if that particular food had never caused her trouble before. Eventually, she had limited her breakfast to a cup of black coffee and two Ritz crackers. Lunch was limited to a turkey sandwich with mustard but without lettuce, tomato, butter, or mayonnaise, a small portion of sorbet, and a cup of black coffee. Dinner was always a piece of skinless chicken and cooked asparagus with mashed potatoes. She ate these same meals day in and day out. All of this, of course, was unnecessary and reflected an underlying emotional disorder and a failure to recognize how to properly test the cause-and-effect relationship for individual food sensitivities. Her psychologist and I encouraged her to experiment with other foods and she gradually added more appetizing and nutritious foods to her diet. Although her symptoms would come and go, she was able to get herself to accept that they were not always directly related to the foods she was eating.

Be sure to note in your journal how much of each item you're eating or drinking. With that information in hand, you can spot ways to make gradual modifications in portion sizes, cut down on fats and spicy foods, and include more non-gassy cooked vegetables in your meals and snacks.

By listing the times you eat throughout the day, you can also uncover other unhealthy patterns. Skipping breakfast and/or lunch and then eating a large meal at the end of a tiring day right before bedtime is a pattern I've seen in many of my patients.

When you stray off your planned eating and exercising regimen, your diary can often help you understand why the lapse happened. In chapter 3, we'll discuss in more detail how to keep a journal and use it to discover patterns of behavior that may be triggering your GI symptoms.

- ***THE DAILY RECORD***
- A journal can help you establish possible links between certain foods and your GI symptoms. Plus, by including the amounts of each of the foods you've eaten, the journal can help you plan ways of gradually cutting down on fats, caffeine, alcohol, and troublesome foods.

10. Watch Out for Non-food "Triggers" That Kick In Your Digestive Symptoms

In addition to tracking food triggers, I recommend that you use your journal to keep an inventory of psychological and social triggers that cause you to overeat or repeatedly induce GI symptoms. For instance, patients with irritable bowel syndrome often experience a flare-up following stressful encounters with difficult bosses, family members, or romantic partners. In trying to avoid this stress, some patients have responded to their GI symptoms by developing extreme lifestyles in which they avoid difficult situations in life. I strongly recommend that you not do this. In chapter 5, I show you how you can live in the real world—not run away from it—by confronting these triggers and learning to manage your symptoms.

One of my patients discovered through keeping a journal that her symptoms worsened every time she had a meeting with her boss. She left the meetings with lots of questions in her mind, "Exactly what does she want me to do?" "Didn't she like the job I did on the last project?" "Doesn't she know how I feel about working on the Smith account?" We discussed ways in which she could improve her communication skills with her boss, and she found that these techniques helped both her and her boss to come away from meetings with a clearer understanding of each other's needs and expectations.

Do you feel your stomach knot up when you hear your in-laws are coming to dinner? Do you feel queasy when you're asked to deliver a report at work? Do social situations like cocktail parties trigger bloating, diarrhea, abdominal pain, or other symptoms? Do you drink pots of coffee and smoke packs of cigarettes when you're working or studying late at night? We'll discuss ways to deal with stress, anxiety, depression, and other triggers that cause you to stray from your healthy eating program in chapter 5.

Now that you're familiar with *The Insider Rules,* you can move on to chapter 3, where we'll discuss a new food pyramid—or eating plan—designed for people suffering from various GI complaints. I encourage you to apply *The Insider Rules* when adopting your new way of eating.

3

Eating Well to Feel Good

....

SN'T it interesting that the biblical history of the human race begins with the choice to eat what is forbidden? The modern world is an Eden of potentially damaging foods, most of which are hard to resist, and the abundance of options can be overwhelming. It seems that we are always wrestling with either what we *want* to eat or what we think we *should* eat. If our motives were based strictly on nutrition, the choices would probably be simple.

As infants, we started with only one choice—our mother's milk. It was nutritious, delicious, and made us feel good. But as we grew, we were given more choices, and eventually those choices became more complicated. Nutrition, health, and feeling good were no longer linked to one perfect food.

As adults, we make food choices based on any number of reasons that have nothing to do with nutrition or health. We eat because we enjoy the act of eating. We eat foods like home-style macaroni and cheese for comfort; we eat foods like steak, lobster, and champagne to display social status; we eat at parties and family gatherings to feel close to others; and sometimes we eat because we are depressed, bored, frustrated, or angry.

I once had a patient named Maria who had gastroesophageal reflux disease and was quite overweight. To help alleviate her heartburn, I had been trying to encourage her to control her overeating, but Maria ate with a vengeance. She and her mother had been engaged in a battle over her weight ever since Maria's childhood. Now every bite was an unconscious blow against her mother. "Take that!" she seemed to be saying as she stuffed in the mashed potatoes. Unfortunately, Maria suffered far more than her mother did as a consequence of her emotional eating. Until she came to grips with all the motives behind her overeating, no diet would solve her problems.

Maria's problem was magnified by the incredible availability of food in our culture. We face an almost infinite number of choices, many of which our great-grandparents might not even have recognized as food. Back then, there were no protein bars, no frozen dinners, no liquid diets, no dehydrated mixes, no sports drinks, no artificial sweeteners.

What did our earliest ancestors eat? Anthropologists believe that they ate a predominantly vegetarian diet with occasional feasts of meat from a successful hunt. By today's standards, food was relatively scarce. Our ancestors were physically active and nearly continuously exposed to the elements. Their bodies were probably lean and muscular, with little accumulation of fat.

During the Neolithic period, humans began to produce food for the first time. They kept livestock and became proficient farmers. Over time, they began to consume dairy products, eggs, cereals, breads, alcoholic beverages, and salt. For the most part, though, complex carbohydrates in the form of grains, bread, potatoes, and beans constituted the bulk of their diet. And, for the majority of people in the world today—those living in other cultures—these foods still supply 60 percent or more of our daily calories.

Our Grandparents Ate Better Than We Do

It is only over the past 150 years or so, in conditions of peace and affluence, that we have turned to high-fat foods of animal origin and refined sugar, salt, and alcohol. Let's take a look at how our eating habits have changed over the years:

- In 1910, Americans were eating 32 percent of their daily calories in the form of fats.
- By 1976, fats made up 42 percent of our daily diets.
- Today, despite grocery store shelves lined with foods touting the labels "low fat," "98% fat-free," and "fat reduced," we still eat a diet made up of close to 40 percent fats.

In our grandparents' day, grains and complex carbohydrates were the mainstay of the America diet. This has changed, too:

- In 1910, carbohydrates from a wide range of whole grains, including rye, barley, buckwheat, and corn, provided 37 percent of people's daily calories.

- In 1976, carbohydrates accounted for only 21 percent of our daily calories.
- Today, they supply just 18 percent of our daily intake.

Another look at the statistics show how our passion for sweets has grown and influenced our diet:

- In 1910, sweeteners supplied only 12 percent of people's daily calories.
- In 1976, refined sugar, corn syrup, and other high-calorie sweeteners made up 18 percent of our calories.
- Today, as many as 25 percent of our calories can come from sweeteners, some largely hidden in prepared foods, such as spaghetti sauce and salad dressings, which we don't consider "sweet."

Prior to the 1940s, the diseases related to the American diet were deficiency diseases, those caused by lack of a necessary nutrient. People who didn't get enough vitamin D developed *rickets,* a condition in which the bones become soft and deformed. People who didn't get enough vitamin C developed *scurvy,* a disease in which the gums become spongy and the teeth begin to loosen. *Pellagra,* a disease that comes from a diet too low in niacin and protein caused skin problems, gastrointestinal disorders, and central nervous system symptoms. People who didn't get enough thiamine suffered from *beri-beri,* which caused nerve, digestive, and heart problems.

Today, instead of seeing many illnesses that are caused by dietary deficiencies, we see far more diseases that are caused by eating too much food or the wrong foods. Our supermarkets are minefields of dangerously calorie- and fat-laden foods that are either easy-to-prepare or ready-to-eat. Fast-food chains—many with drive-through service—make it far too easy for us to pick up high-fat, high-calorie meals on the way home from a hard day at work. We're not even safe within our own homes—where advertisers bombard us with entertaining television commercials that make us crave "junk" foods we see on the screen by showing happy, healthy people enjoying them.

AVOID FAD DIETS

Have you considered going on one of the popular high-protein, low-carbohydrate, high-fat diets that are all the rage these days, such as the Atkins and Eades diets? I advise my patients to avoid these fad diets, as many experts don't consider them very healthful, and in my experience, they make GI problems worse. Eating a diet high in fat has been shown to increase the risk of many types of cancer, including colon cancer (cancer of the large part of the intestine). For patients who have heartburn, a high intake of fats promotes reflux by reducing the pressure of the lower esophageal sphincter. The best way to get the proper balance of fats, proteins, carbohydrates, and other nutrients is to follow the "Food Guide Pyramid" in this chapter, personalizing it to take into consideration your own special dietary needs.

It's no wonder that so many of my patients today—especially those with heartburn—have been in the habit of making poor food choices. When I first meet patients whose dietary choices apparently have been driven more by what "sounds good" than by what's truly good for them, I give them a blueprint to guide their eating choices. It's called the Food Guide Pyramid. Let's take a look at how it works.

Getting the Right Balance of Foods

Diets that are high in fat and contain more calories than the body uses are out of balance. So are diets that are low in grain products, vegetables, fruit, and fiber. Healthful diets contain the appropriate amounts of nutrients and calories needed to prevent nutritional deficiencies and excesses. They provide the right balance of carbohydrate, fat, and protein. But eating a balanced diet requires thought and careful consideration, rather than choosing foods that simply "sound good." Some foods, such as grain products, vegetables, and fruits, have many nutrients and other healthful substances but are relatively low in calories. Fat and alcohol are high in calories. Foods high in both sugars and fat contain many calories but are often low in vitamins, minerals, or fiber.

The Food Guide Pyramid is a food-ranking system developed by the U.S. Department of Agriculture (USDA) in 1992 to capture in a visually simple manner the basic five food groups and number of recommended daily servings for the average person. The pyramid starts with grains at the bottom layer (6–11 servings), then the vegetable group (3–5 servings) and fruit group (2–4 servings) on the next layer, then dairy (2–3 servings) and meat/poultry/fish/dried beans/eggs/nuts (2–3 servings) on the next layer.

It's important to understand what is meant by a "serving." Here are some examples of what counts as a serving in each of the food groups:

The USDA Food Guide Pyramid

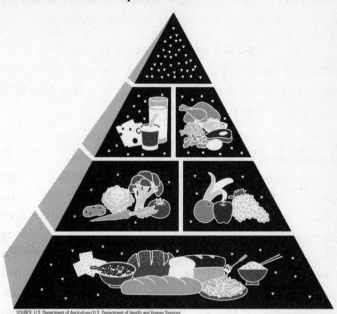

SOURCE: U.S. Department of Agriculture/U.S. Department of Health and Human Services

- Grain products: 1 slice of bread; ½ cup of rice, pasta, or cooked cereal (choose whole grains whenever possible).
- Vegetables: 1 cup of raw leafy vegetables; ½ cup of other chopped or cooked vegetables.
- Fruits: 1 medium orange, apple, banana; ½ cup of chopped, cooked, or canned fruit; ¾ cup of fruit juice.
- Dairy products: 1 cup of milk or yogurt; 1½ ounces of natural cheese. Be sure to choose low-fat or nonfat varieties of all dairy products.
- Meat, fish, poultry, eggs, beans, nuts: 2–3 ounces of cooked lean meat, poultry, or fish; ½ cup of cooked

dry beans. One egg, 2 tablespoons of peanut butter, or ⅓ cup of nuts is equivalent to 1 ounce of meat.

SIZING UP YOUR SERVINGS

If you're like many Americans today, you may have lost sight of proper-size portions of foods. Here are some simple guidelines for estimating the size of a single serving:

Food	One Serving
Cooked vegetables	½ cup, or the size of a small fist
Cooked lean meat, poultry, or fish	2 to 3 ounces, or the size of a deck of playing cards
Bread	One slice, the size of the palm of your hand
Cooked or canned fruit (chopped)	½ cup, or the size of a small fist
Baked potato	½ potato, the size of a computer mouse
Egg	One egg, or ¼ cup egg substitute
Breakfast cereal	1 ounce, or a large handful

Although the Food Guide Pyramid is not an exact science, it's a good starting place for creating a healthful, well-balanced diet. Whole-grain products, vegetables, and fruits are emphasized in the Food Guide Pyramid because they provide vitamins, minerals, complex carbohydrates (starch and dietary fiber), and other substances that are important for good health. They are also generally low in fat—depending on how they are prepared and what is added to them at the table—and they are good for "filling you up." Most Americans eat fewer than the recommended number of servings of grain products, vegetables, and fruits. Those foods in the middle of the pyramid (dairy products and meats) are to be eaten moderately. Most people consume far too much from the top tier of the pyramid, the space reserved for fats, oils, and sweets, which should be consumed only sparingly.

GO WITH THE GRAIN

When choosing breads and cereals, look for whole-grain varieties, including whole wheat, cracked wheat, and multigrain. For the healthiest bread, read the label: "Stone ground whole wheat flour" (not "enriched wheat flour") should be listed as the first ingredient, which means that it is made from 100 percent whole-wheat flour and is not just a blend of refined white and wheat flours. Check the labels whenever you buy breads and cereals; look for those made of "whole grain" and have at least 2 grams of fiber per serving. (Label-reading hint: The first ingredient listed is the one with the greatest amount in the product.) When buying rice, choose brown rice over white rice. Experiment with other cooked grains such as oats, barley, rye, quinoa, and kamut.

Foods within each group of the pyramid supply similar nutrients. By eating the suggested number of servings from each group, you automatically eat a balanced diet. Because each food group contains a variety of foods, it's easy to find a number of healthful choices that appeal to your taste. However, for the average person who suffers from heartburn, gas, bloating, constipation, diarrhea, or stomach pain, certain foods within the various food groups can be troublesome and should be avoided. That means that you'll want to choose other foods within that same food group instead of those that trigger or worsen digestive symptoms—so that your overall diet remains in proper balance.

FIBER FACTS

Fiber is a mix of many different kinds of plant material that is not digested and absorbed in the small intestine. Eating a diet with plenty of high-fiber foods—whole grains, whole-grain breads and cereals, vegetables, and fruits—may have several health benefits, including lowering cholesterol and helping protect against heart disease and colon cancer. Eating fiber-rich foods can also make you feel fuller longer and contribute to weight control. Most important for patients with digestive problems, however, fiber helps avoid constipation and is an aid to some people with irritable bowel syndrome.

Fiber is generally divided into two categories: *soluble fiber* dissolves in water and *insoluble fiber* is like a sponge and cannot dissolve in water. Soluble fiber is found in oats, oat bran, seeds, brown rice, dried beans and peas, barley vegetables (such as carrots, corn, cauliflower, and sweet potatoes), and fruits (such as apples, strawberries, oranges, bananas, nectarines, and pears). It can help soften stools. Insoluble fiber is found in wheat bran, corn bran, whole-wheat breads and cereals, vegetables (such as potatoes with skin, parsnips, green beans, and broccoli), and fruits. It helps increase stool bulk and may reduce the symptoms of some digestive disorders.

As you can see, some foods (mainly fruits and vegetables) contain both soluble and insoluble fiber. While fruits and vegetables are good sources of fiber whether they are served raw or cooked, I recommend that my patients who have gas or bloating always eat their fruits and vegetables thoroughly *cooked.* During the cooking process, chemical bonds in the fruits and vegetables are broken, releasing hydrogen gas in the cooking pan instead of in the patient's digestive tract, which helps reduce gas and bloating. Some of my patients who can tolerate eating spices have reported that adding garlic, ginger, or nutmeg to vegetables or fruits in cooking helps alleviate gas, as these spices help break down gas-causing components as well.

The key to adding fiber to your diet is to add it gradually. If you suddenly boost the fiber content of your diet, you might experience unnecessary abdominal pain, diarrhea, and/or gas. As you add fiber to your diet, drink plenty of fluids and eat as many unprocessed foods as you can, choosing whole grain foods, eating the skin of fruits and vegetables (wash them thoroughly first), and the seeds in fruits such as raspberries and figs. I recommend that my patients get their fiber from foods, not supplements, to reap the full benefits.

Top 20 Fiber-Rich Foods
- 100% bran cereal
- Corn bran cereal
- Lentils
- Chick peas (garbanzo beans)
- Kidney beans
- Green peas
- Winter squash
- Broccoli
- Brussels sprouts
- Blackberries
- Strawberries
- Raspberries
- Prunes
- Figs, dried
- Apricots
- Turnip greens
- Barley
- Sweet potato
- Carrots
- Spinach

I can make many suggestions to the individual GI sufferer about how to adapt the Food Guide Pyramid to meet his or her unique nutritional and physiological needs. For many people with digestive disorders, eating a proper diet lessens their symptoms; however, reworking a diet to alleviate or eliminate a GI condition requires more than the elimination of junk food. Even certain healthy foods can aggravate the systems of those with heartburn, gas, bloating, constipation, diarrhea, or stomach pain. For example, cabbage, broccoli, and beans are healthful, nutritious foods for most people, but people who suffer from gas and bloating cannot tolerate them—especially when they are served raw instead of thoroughly cooked—because these foods produce gas in the digestive tract. In the same way, low-fat or nonfat milk and milk products are healthful sources of protein and calcium for most people, but those who are lactose-intolerant should avoid them or use special enzyme supplements, such as Lactaid, to help break down milk sugars.

In this chapter I'll show you how to use your food journal to create your own personal food guide pyramid that will help you eat a balanced diet and quell your unique set of GI symptoms. And I'll give you tips for getting started in making changes to your diet in ways that don't disrupt your status quo too much.

At the end of this chapter, I'll provide food lists of do's and don'ts suited to each of the common digestive symptoms, based on what has worked for many other people who experienced them. Every person is unique, however, and I found the best way to determine your individual list of symptom-inducing foods and behaviors is to use your journal.

LACTOSE INTOLERANCE

If you have trouble digesting milk and milk products, you may have a condition known as *lactose intolerance*. Lactose is a large sugar molecule found in milk products. People who are lactose-intolerant lack an enzyme called lactase that normally helps people digest this molecule before it reaches the intestines, where it causes gas, cramps, bloating, and diarrhea.

If dairy products cause your symptoms to flare up, obviously your first recourse is to eat less of those foods. You may tolerate yogurt better because it contains organisms that supply lactase. If you choose to avoid dairy products, be sure to substitute other foods that contain calcium (such as soy products) or calcium supplements. Most people need between 1200 and 1500 milligrams of calcium daily. Try these non-dairy sources:

- Calcium-fortified orange or apple juice, cereals, and soy milk
- Almonds, sunflower seeds, and pistachios
- Broccoli, Brussels sprouts, and cauliflower
- Kale, mustard greens, and spinach

You can also look for lactose-reduced milk and cheeses in your grocer's dairy case. They are available in low-fat and nonfat varieties. Special enzyme supplements are also widely available to help you digest milk sugar. Look for these under the brand names Lactaid, Lactrase, and DairyEase. Some of these products come in tablet form that you take before eating a dairy-containing meal. Others are drops that you put in milk before you drink it.

A WORD ABOUT SALT

Salt, or sodium (one of the components of salt), can cause water retention (fluid buildup) in some people. Sometimes people refer to this fluid buildup as "bloating." When I talk about bloating here or with my patients, I mean the buildup of air or gas in the digestive tract, which is not affected by eating salt or sodium. Although eating too much sodium (the American Heart Association recommends less than 2000 milligrams daily) doesn't affect gastrointestinal disorders, it's not good for overall health. Eating too much sodium can increase blood pressure in some people and should be avoided by anyone with heart trouble or kidney failure.

Many Americans consume too much sodium—not because they shake too much salt on their food at the table, but because of the hidden sodium in processed foods. You expect sodium in your potato chips or pickles, but you'll be surprised at how much is in that jar of spaghetti sauce. Read the labels on the packaged foods you buy (the key word is *sodium,* not just "salt") to see how much sodium they contain, and look for reduced-sodium products, such as broths, soups, crackers, cheese, and ham. When cooking, use lemon, fresh or dried herbs, and spices instead of salt to intensify flavors.

Keeping a Journal

As we learned in chapter 2, it's a good idea to keep a journal noting which foods seem to cause distress before you begin changing your diet. A journal can help you establish possible links between certain foods and your GI symptoms. By keeping a record of everything you eat, what time of day you ate it, and how you felt before, during, and after eating it, you can begin to get a clearer picture of your current eating patterns. You'll begin to see which foods cause the most digestive problems and how healthful your overall diet really is.

To make your journal most useful for detecting what helps and what hurts your gut, you'll need to record *everything* you eat and drink. By recording each food immediately after you eat it, you'll be less likely to forget to include everything. Remember, every mouthful of food "tested" while you were cooking dinner and every snack you ate standing at the kitchen sink should be recorded, too, as should chewing gum and candy.

Besides writing down *what* you ate (the specific food and how it was prepared, such as "fried chicken" or "broiled salmon"), record *when* (the time of day) each food or beverage was consumed, as well as *where* you were (such as in the kitchen at home, at a restaurant, in the car, or in your office) when you ate or drank it. Record *how much* of the food you ate (1 cup, 16 ounces, etc.). Then write down whether you were alone or with someone else (name them) and any activity (such as watching television, playing cards, surfing the Internet, or reading a book) that you were doing while you were eating or drinking. Finally, write down how you were feeling when you ate. Were you happy, sad, bored, tired, or in a rush?

See the sample day's journal on pages 86–87.

How to Analyze Your Journal

After you have compiled a week or two of daily journals, it's time to sit down (either alone or with your doctor or a

PERSONAL FOOD JOURNAL

When did I eat or drink?	Where was I when I ate or drank it?	What did I eat or drink?	How much did I have?	What else was I doing?	Who was with me?	How was I feeling?
6:15 A.M.	Kitchen	Coffee Ham Swiss cheese	2 cups 1 slice (1 oz) ½ slice (1 oz)	Packing lunch; unloading the dishwasher	No one	Worried about the meeting at work; constipated; worried about being constipated
8:30 A.M.	Next to the coffeepot at the office	Coffee Doughnut (glazed)	1 cup 1 doughnut	Talking with coworkers	Mary, Jim, Sue	Worried about the meeting; stomach hurts; diarrhea

Time	Location	Food	Amount	Activity	With Whom	Mood
12:30 P.M.	At my desk	Ham and Swiss cheese sandwich (mustard, mayonnaise, lettuce, tomato) on sourdough bread; potato chips, Coke	1 sandwich 8 oz. chips 12 oz. drink	Writing up my notes from the meeting	No one	Happy that the meeting went so well
3:00 P.M.	Next to the coffeepot at the office	Chocolate fudge cake	1 large slice	Celebrating Sue's birthday	Whole office staff	Happy, laughing, feeling good
8:00 P.M.	In the living room	Double-cheese pizza Red wine	2 large slices 2 glasses	Watching TV	No one	Tired, bored
11:30 P.M.	In bed	Cognac	2 oz. glass	Reading	No one	Lonely

nutritionist) and analyze your eating patterns. Do you eat a good variety and balance of foods? What proportions of your daily diet come from carbohydrates, proteins, fats, and empty-calorie foods (such as sugar and alcohol)? Do you grab junk food when you're in a hurry? How often do you eat fresh fruits and vegetables? We'll discuss how emotions can trigger digestive symptoms in chapter 5, but keep in mind that your mood can also influence your eating behavior. If your journal unveils that you overeat—or that you eat certain foods you know are unhealthful—you can take steps to deal with your moods in more appropriate ways.

The patient who prepared the journal in the example was clearly consuming far too much fat, sugar, salt, and alcohol—and not nearly enough complex carbohydrates. When we went over her journal entries, she was surprised at how many cups of coffee she was drinking and how much fat she was consuming. As she collected several days' entries, we were able to begin to discern certain eating patterns that contributed to her weight problem and caused her uncomfortable digestive symptoms to worsen.

Sometimes food diaries help people understand their symptoms in unexpected ways. For example, a twenty-nine-year-old woman who was a successful junior executive in a large multinational company had experienced lifelong good health, but for the past year, diarrhea had become a frequent problem. When I questioned her, she said she had not experienced many of the usual symptoms of irritable bowel syndrome, such as gas, bloating, constipation alternating with diarrhea, abdominal crampy pain, or rumbling and gurgling in the abdomen. Despite the fact she hadn't experienced any symptoms other than diarrhea, I still suspected she had irritable bowel syndrome. We often refer to this condition as "diarrhea-predominant irritable bowel syndrome."

She had seen two excellent gastroenterologists and had undergone a thorough, extensive evaluation that included colonoscopy, upper endoscopy, small bowel X-ray, and stool cultures for bacteria as well as for parasites. Results from a panel of blood tests were totally normal. Nothing seemed to be wrong—except that she was experiencing diarrhea several times a day on most days.

I questioned her about her diet and she told me that she was quite careful to eat a balanced diet and to limit her intake of fat and calories. She had been weight-conscious throughout her adult life and had struggled to keep her weight under good control.

PUT IT IN WRITING

Merely by keeping a journal, you'll find that your eating habits will improve. Jotting down what you eat makes you more aware of your food choices. Sometimes, just because you know you'll have to record it, you'll find yourself saying no to high-fat and sugar-laden snacks. Plus, your journal will help you be honest with yourself. That extra helping of dessert you ate in the kitchen when no one else was looking still "counts" when you have to include it in your journal.

To try to determine what was causing her diarrhea, I asked her to keep a food journal and to be sure to record everything she put in her mouth. She brought her diary in in about two weeks. I reviewed the foods she had eaten and didn't see any listed that should trigger diarrhea. However, I noticed that several times each day she was in the habit of chewing sugar-free gum. She hadn't mentioned the gum when we had discussed her diet earlier, and she hadn't thought it worth mentioning to her previous doctors, either. The gum was sweetened with sorbitol, a substance that can cause severe diarrhea in some people.

I recommended that she avoid the chewing gum containing sorbitol, and within seventy-two hours, her diarrhea stopped, never to return. Only because she was careful to write down *everything* she put into her mouth in her journal were we able to detect the culprit that had been causing her diarrhea.

HEARTBURN VS. GAS

When being a diet detective, it's important to recognize that some symptoms take longer to show up than others. For example, heartburn usually occurs shortly (usually within minutes, not hours) after eating an offending food. Gas, however, might be noted minutes after eating a gas-producing food, or it might not show up for hours, until the food has made its way through the digestive tract and is being broken down by bacteria in the large intestine (colon). Keep these facts in mind when examining your food journal. Gas you experience in the evening might be caused by something you ate for lunch or by something you ate for dinner. On the other hand, heartburn in the evening is more likely to have been triggered by a food you ate for dinner than by one you ate hours ago for lunch.

Clues to Look For in Your Journal Entries

As you review your journal entries, keep in mind that while you're unique and have your own set of foods that trigger symptoms, it's likely that some of the foods other people have found troublesome will turn out to be symptom-inducers for you as well. Here are some foods that many people with irritable bowel syndrome have found problematic:

- High-fat, fried, or greasy foods. Fats slow down the digestive tract, gumming up the works in your system.
- Gas-forming foods, such as cabbage, broccoli, cauliflower, coleslaw (which is made from cabbage), corn, beans, nuts, and carbonated beverages. If you experience excess gassiness, you may find it helpful to eliminate these foods from your diet for a while. They may be reintroduced once your symptoms have gone away. (See sidebar on the "Top Ten Gas-Producing Foods.")
- Fresh fruits or fructose (found in fruits and dates)
- Beverages that contain caffeine (coffee, black tea, cola, chocolate)
- Decaffeinated coffee
- Milk and milk products (if you are lactose-intolerant)
- Bubbly (carbonated) beverages, including seltzer water, soft drinks, and beer
- Foods containing sorbitol, such as diet candies and gum. (See sidebar "Mints, Gum, Tums, and Rolaids" on page 94 for more information.)
- Bran cereals. Bran products may help some people but others cannot tolerate them.

READ LABELS

I don't necessarily suggest to tally up their daily total of fat grams that my patients carry around a fat gram table. But I do recommend that they check food labels for fat content and that they avoid fat-laden foods such as whole milk products, butter, oils, salad dressings, and fried foods.

BEWARE OF HIDDEN SOURCES OF FAT IN FOODS

- Think you're choosing wisely by selecting the fish sandwich at a fast-food restaurant? They often contain more fat than hamburgers. If the restaurant posts nutrition information, read it before you order.

- Test foods such as crackers, muffins, or cookies for fat content by setting them on a sheet of brown grocer's paper or a paper towel. If they leave a greasy residue on the paper, they contain too much fat.

- Think you need to pour a little cooking oil in your pan for sautéing? Try using nonfat cooking sprays and/or non-stick pans instead. If you insist on using cooking oil, put it in a spray bottle (some gourmet stores now sell special misters for this purpose) and spritz it on lightly, or paint on a thin layer with a pastry brush.

- Avoid pasta covered with oil- or cream-based sauces. Choose tomato-based sauces such as marinara instead.

- If the salad bar chicken is glistening, beware! That shiny surface is a dead giveaway that it has been prepared with oil.

- Always read labels. That "healthy" soy drink might be loaded with fat grams.

TOP TEN GAS-PRODUCING FOODS

- Cabbage
- Cauliflower
- Broccoli
- Brussels sprouts
- Turnips
- Dried beans
- Onions
- Garlic
- Leeks
- Milk products (in patients who lack the enzyme lactase)

Dried beans are perhaps the most well-known gas producers. They cause gas and flatulence even in people who don't normally have trouble with gas and bloating. It's not so much the beans themselves that produce the gas, but their skins. The bean skins pass into the large intestine (colon) undigested, where intestinal bacteria break their carbohydrates into sugars, releasing gas in the process. Many people believe that soaking the dried beans in water for 12 to 24 hours, discarding the water, and rinsing the beans thoroughly before cooking helps eliminate much of the gas, as soaking helps break down the carbohydrates in the bean skins. I have not, however, found this to produce a major difference in my patients who have serious trouble with gas and bloating.

Some find that a few drops of Beano, a special enzyme supplement available in drugstores and health food stores, helps alleviate gas when added to precooked beans.

- *SIP DON'T GULP*
- If gas is a problem for you, you may want to examine your
- drinking habits. It seems that people swallow more air with
- drinks than with foods. You're likely to swallow even more
- air when drinking through a straw or from a bottle or can
- than from a glass. Try to sip slowly instead of gulping; you'll
- swallow less air that way.

MINTS, GUM, TUMS, AND ROLAIDS

Many of my patients have adopted the habit of popping mints, gums, candies, and mint-flavored antacids like Tums and Rolaids into their mouths throughout the day. This really isn't a good idea. Any kind of mint (peppermint, wintergreen, or spearmint) will reduce the lower esophageal pressure and allow more reflux in patients who get heartburn.

Tums and its equivalents are calcium-containing antacids. Because of the calcium, taking Tums too often may lead to constipation. If you're taking Tums or Rolaids all day long, you're probably doing so because you're not getting relief from your symptoms. In some cases, you may be better off taking a more potent prescription drug for a while if the measures in this book don't work for you. Neither Tums nor Rolaids are as potent as prescription drugs (such as proton-pump inhibitors).

If you can't break your gum habit and sorbitol gives you diarrhea, look for gums that contain other sugars like xylitol or sugar substitutes such as saccharin, which are not known to cause diarrhea.

SMALLER IS BETTER

Large meals can cause cramping and diarrhea in people with irritable bowel syndrome. Symptoms may be eased if you eat smaller meals more often or if you just eat smaller portions. This should help, especially if your meals are low in fat and high in carbohydrates such as pasta, rice, whole-grain breads and cereals, fruits and vegetables.

DIARRHEA DEMONS

Diarrhea can occur as a result of infection with a virus, bacteria, or parasite. Diarrhea (often preceded by vomiting) can also result from food poisoning. These kinds of bouts with diarrhea are generally over in a day or two. Diarrhea that's associated with a digestive disorder (such as irritable bowel syndrome) occurs whenever a person eats certain trigger foods or is experiencing stress. In people who experience diarrhea due to irritable bowel syndrome, here are some of the common food offenders:

Top Food-Related Diarrhea Demons

- Sorbitol (in sorbitol-sensitive people)
- Prune juice or other fruit juices
- Unpeeled fruits, such as apples, grapes, plums, or pears
- Milk products (in people who lack the enzyme lactase)
- Fatty or fried foods
- Caffeine (coffee, chocolate, colas)
- Raw vegetables, such as in those coleslaw or salads

Top Diarrhea Fighters

- The BRAT foods (bananas, rice, apples or applesauce, toast)
- Lactaid (in people who are lactose intolerant)

CAFFEINE CONTENT OF VARIOUS FOODS AND OVER-THE-COUNTER MEDICINES

Item	Amount	Caffeine (milligrams)
Drip coffee	7 ounces	115 to 175
Brewed coffee	7 ounces	80 to 135
Instant coffee	7 ounces	65 to 100
Espresso	7 ounces	100
Starbucks coffee grande	16 ounces	550
Decaf coffee, brewed	7 ounces	3 to 4
Decaf coffee, instant	7 ounces	2 to 3
Hot chocolate	8 ounces	5
Tea, brewed	7 ounces	40 to 60
Tea, instant	7 ounces	30
Tea, iced	12 ounces	70
Coca-Cola (diet or regular)	12 ounces	46
Pepsi Cola	12 ounces	37
Jolt Cola	12 ounces	71
Mountain Dew	12 ounces	55
7-Up (diet or regular)	12 ounces	0
Chocolate milk	8 ounces	5
Cadbury chocolate bar	1 ounce	15
Hershey chocolate bar	1.5 ounces	10
Häagen-Dazs coffee ice cream	1 cup	58
No-Doz, maximum strength or Vivarin	1 tablet	200
No-Doz, regular strength	1 tablet	100
Excedrin	2 tablets	130
Anacin	2 tablets	64

People who experience heartburn or acid indigestion should look for other possible triggers when examining their journals:

• High-fat foods tend to make heartburn worse. Watch out for the one-two punch: fatty foods are especially a problem when consumed quickly and along with carbonated drinks, alcohol, or coffee. This explains why a typical fast-food meal on the run consisting of a hamburger, french fries, and cola can trigger heartburn symptoms in many people.

• Large-volume meals can trigger heartburn. It's also a good idea to stop eating three or four hours before you go to bed to give the acid in the stomach a chance to decrease and the stomach to empty partially.

• Certain foods can weaken the LES (the one-way valve that keeps stomach contents from backing up into the esophagus). These foods include chocolate, mints (such as peppermint, wintergreen, and spearmint), fatty foods, coffee, and alcohol. Foods that can irritate a damaged esophageal lining, such as citrus fruits and juices, tomato products, and pepper, should also be avoided.

Your journal can also help you separate *true* food-triggered symptoms from those that are unrelated to the food you ate. Remember the patient with irritable bowel syndrome in chapter 2 who trusted her memory instead of keeping a journal? Whenever she would experience unpleasant digestive symptoms, she would recall what food she had eaten recently and would then eliminate that food from her diet—even if that particular food had never caused her trouble before. Eventually, she had limited herself to a mere handful of foods that she believed she could tolerate. The problem was, she didn't know how to properly test the cause-and-effect relationship for individual food sensitivities.

- ***KNOW YOUR TRIGGERS***
- When you've experienced a symptom such as heartburn
- after eating, it's far more likely that the offending food is one
- that frequently causes heartburn in other people as well. By
- referring to the lists of food triggers discussed in this book,
- you can avoid unnecessarily eliminating "innocent" foods
- from your diet.

Jumping to the wrong conclusions about food "culprits" and then unnecessarily eliminating them from a diet is a problem I see all the time among my patients. Jeaninne was a woman in her fifties who had experienced uncomfortable symptoms associated with irritable bowel syndrome for most of her adult life. While raising two children, she managed to advance in her career from an entry-level job as a file clerk to a demanding position as an executive administrative assistant—in spite of her symptoms, which included alternating diarrhea and constipation as well as intermittent abdominal cramps. For many years, these symptoms had appeared in the afternoon or early evening, but Jeaninne had always been able to spend most of the evening in comfort and rarely would lose any sleep because of them. During the past year, however, she found that her sleep was often being interrupted by gas, bloating, rumbling, gurgling, and abdominal swelling, which generally started around bedtime and made it difficult for her to fall asleep. Then, once she did fall asleep, she was restless and sometimes would even wake up because of the discomfort she felt from the gas and swelling.

Jeaninne knew that she wouldn't be able to function well at her job if she kept having trouble sleeping, so she tried to figure out what was causing her nighttime symptoms. For many years, one of the few dietary pleasures she allowed herself was eating a few sugar cookies before bedtime. Because of the onset of her abdominal gas, bloating, rumbling, and gurgling around the time when she would eat her nightly sugar cookies, she decided that this pleasurable food must be responsible for her symptoms, and she eliminated them from her diet.

Yet Jeaninne's symptoms failed to improve. I asked her to bring in a diet journal. It was clear from it that she had enjoyed her sugar cookies for quite some time, but she had recently introduced a lot of vegetables, such as broccoli and Brussels sprouts, into her diet. She thought that this was acceptable because they were well cooked, and she believed only raw vegetables would cause gas. I suggested that she eliminate them from her diet and see what happened to her symptoms. She did so and within a few days her nighttime gas and bloating had gone away. Besides being relieved of her uncomfortable symptoms, she was once again able to allow herself the pleasure of enjoying a couple of sugar cookies before she went to bed. Her symptoms have not recurred.

It's All in the Details

The more detailed your diet journal is, the better it can help you determine exactly which foods are triggering your symptoms. If you experienced symptoms after eating a meal consisting of a cheeseburger with fries and a Coke, say, it's a good bet that the high-fat content of the meal contributed to your problem, but it's harder to tell if you're sensitive to dairy products (the cheese) or to caffeine (in the Coke). In fact, it may be the onions, tomatoes, or mustard on the burger or the large amount of ketchup you poured generously over the fries. That's why it's important to list every ingredient you can for each dish, including condiments like mustard, relish, mayonnaise, ketchup, and sauerkraut, and to record every mouthful you eat from morning to night. One of my patients, a well-to-do business executive who traveled frequently, discovered that the chocolate-covered mints his five-star hotel provided on his pillow at night—wrapped in fancy gold foil—were contributing to his nighttime heartburn. He had almost neglected to include them in his journal because they were so small he considered them insignificant.

Amounts or serving sizes—whether they're small or large—are important to record as well. For many of my patients, *how much* they eat is as much of a problem as *what* they eat. I've noticed that sometimes my patients can tolerate a tiny amount of a certain food, but they experience symptoms when they consume that same food in larger amounts. Be sure to note in your journal how much of each item you're eating or drinking. With that information in hand, you can spot ways to make gradual modifications in portion sizes, cut down on fats and spicy foods, or include more non-gassy cooked vegetables in your meals and snacks. You may need to do some measuring or weighing (there are many inexpensive, easy-to-use kitchen scales) for a while until you can accurately "eyeball" a serving size.

Restaurants tend to offer hefty portions, and many Americans have lost sight of what a normal portion of food is. It is especially important to learn to estimate appropriate portion sizes of foods that may contribute significant amounts of fat to your diet, such as meats, dairy products, dressings, butter, margarine, and cooking oils. Read the labels on packaged foods to check the serving size. You could easily be consuming double or triple the suggested serving size.

A forty-eight-year-old longtime friend of mine named Roger came to see me as a patient because of his concern that recurrent heartburn might lead to cancer of the esophagus. He had experienced heartburn for about three years, but recently he had seen an ad that warned that gastroesophageal reflux disease, if left untreated, could result in the growth of cells that line the stomach over the surface of the lower third of the esophagus. These sensitive cells, when subjected to the constant irritation of acid reflux can, on occasion, become malignant and lead to cancer of the esophagus. Until Roger saw that advertisement, he had not really been concerned about his heartburn. For him, it was a bothersome, but not incapacitating, condition. Because I had known Roger for many years, I was aware that he had experienced a progressive and significant increase in weight during the past four years. Although his weight had fluctuated throughout his life, it had been under control in large part due to an exercise program, until he discontinued it several years ago. Since dropping his daily jogging habit, he had progressively gained weight—at a rate of about ten to fifteen pounds per year—and, as his weight increased, his heartburn worsened.

I explained to Roger that being overweight increases the pressure on the LES (the one-way valve that keeps stomach contents from seeping back up into the esophagus and causing heartburn). I told him that there was a good possibility that with weight loss he could reduce the amount of acid reflux, improve his general sense of well-being, overcome his distressing symptom, and avoid sliding into other medical complications of obesity. He went on a high-protein and low-fat diet, but after two months he was discouraged, because he hadn't lost any significant weight.

I asked him to keep a food diary and to indicate the sizes of his portions in it. When he brought his journal to me for review, his distribution of foods seemed quite appropriate. I noted, though, that he had a difficult time assessing how much of each food he was eating—he often left that column in his food diary blank or simply wrote in "one serving."

One night I had dinner with Roger and his wife at their home, and it then became clear to me that what Roger considered an average portion was enough to feed two or three people. We had a long discussion about portion sizes, and we also discussed the concept of satisfying the taste buds with a small amount of well-prepared food instead of getting stuffed on large quantities of food that you hardly even taste as it goes down.

He listened and agreed that his diet wasn't going to work until he could learn to control his portion sizes. He began a program of actually measuring and weighing his foods, and diligently recorded portion sizes in his diary. His wife, Joyce, helped him out by taping pictures of actual "serving sizes" (which she had found in an article on nutrition in their local newspaper) on the front of their refrigerator door. This helped him begin to recognize that a serving of meat should be about the size of his fist—and not the size of his dinner plate.

At my suggestion, he began experimenting with the concept of simply cutting the portions he would normally eat in half. He jokingly called it his "two-for-one" plan because he and his wife were now going to their favorite restaurants and ordering the same meal they had always enjoyed, except that now they ordered only one dinner and asked for an extra plate so they could share it. At home, they prepared the same amounts of food they used to, and then packaged half of each dinner for freezing so they could have homemade TV dinners another night. Using the "two-for-one" method, he (and, by the way, his wife) started to lose weight.

WEIGHING IN

Many of my patients have had difficulty telling when they've got too much on their plate. Most people are surprised to learn, for example, that one serving of bread is one slice; one serving of chicken is a piece the size of a deck of cards; or one serving of pasta is one cup. If you have trouble estimating food quantities at first, spend some time measuring and weighing your portions until you are sure you can estimate serving sizes by eye. (Food scales are available in gourmet cooking stores and some supermarkets, but you should have one at home, too—even postage scales will work.) When weighing portions, weigh an empty plate, then place the food on the plate and subtract the difference to get the weight of your portion. See the sidebar "Sizing Up Your Servings" earlier in this chapter for more hints on appropriate serving sizes.

After he had lost some weight, he agreed to begin an exercise program, after which he found that he was able to lose weight more rapidly. Once he had lost about forty-five pounds, his self-image greatly improved, as did his general sense of well-being and heartburn.

By listing the times you eat throughout the day, you can also uncover other unhealthy patterns. Skipping breakfast and/or lunch and then eating a large meal at the end of a tiring day right before bedtime is a pattern I've seen in many of my patients. This is an especially bad habit for people who suffer from nighttime heartburn. Bedtime snacks are another unhealthful eating habit that can lead to acid reflux.

In many cases, I believe that it's not just what you eat but when and where and how we eat that affects GI health. I think we were meant to eat three moderate-sized meals a day and once we go beyond that, many of us tend to get into trouble. It's also a good idea to eat sitting down in a comfortable, stress-free setting. Too many people eat on the run—standing in the kitchen by the sink, at their desks at the office, in front of the television set, or even in their cars while driving down the freeway.

For example, I take care of a man in his late thirties who experienced lifelong good health. Throughout his married life his dietary history was quite reasonable and his general health was good. Then he and his wife divorced, and he moved into a bachelor apartment. Following the divorce, he turned even more of his attention to his work and became a greater workaholic than ever. He developed a habit of skipping meals and eating on the run. Frequently, he would work long hours and come home to his empty apartment after 9:00 P.M. Then, tired and lonely, he would eat a large high-fat meal that he had purchased on the way home from one of several fast-food outlets on his route. Following this heavy meal, he would immediately go to bed.

After a few months of this routine, he began experiencing a bitter taste in his mouth upon rising in the morning, and started having frequent episodes of heartburn throughout the day. He paid little attention to his symptoms, and later that year he had several episodes of laryngitis and recurrent bouts of coughing. He eventually came to see me because of the severity of his heartburn. It was difficult to elicit the history described above, but eventually it all came out. As I reviewed with him his dietary history during his married life and his dietary history and lifestyle changes since that time, he realized that his food habits had changed considerably.

CHANGE FOR THE LONG TERM

One of the most common recommendations I make to overweight patients, especially those who experience heartburn, is that they lose weight. To aid them in this endeavor, I help each patient tailor a weight-loss strategy that will work best for him or her. While exercise is a major part of any weight-loss program (discussed in chapter 4), long-term dietary changes are crucial to success. I always point out to patients that they're not "going on a diet," which implies that there will be a time when they "go off their diet." Instead, I ask them to make dietary changes that they can stick with for the rest of their life.

I talked with him about the importance of avoiding large meals and stressed the importance of not reclining for about three hours after eating. I encouraged him to begin an exercise program and to start eating three moderate-sized, well-balanced meals per day. Within a few weeks, all of his symptoms resolved, including his heartburn, bitter taste, laryngitis, and cough. All of these symptoms resulted from acid reflux, which had been exacerbated by stress and eating habits that included a large fatty meal shortly before reclining at night.

Create Your Own Food Guide Pyramid

After you've kept your journal for several weeks, you'll begin to figure out which foods are troublesome for you. But simply eliminating these foods from your diet isn't enough. It's important to use the information you've garnered from your journal to create a personalized version of the basic food guide pyramid just for you. That way, you'll be getting the right balance of nutrients and calories but will be avoiding foods that aggravate your gastrointestinal symptoms. Let's take a look at how one of my patients did this:

Jennifer was a twenty-eight-year-old patient with irritable bowel syndrome who had experienced frequent diarrhea, gas, and bloating before she began trying to make lifestyle modifications. After keeping a detailed journal over a period of several weeks, Jennifer was able to determine that salads made from raw vegetables, especially coleslaw, triggered her gas and bloating. I recommended that she try eating only well-cooked vegetables. She found that green beans, carrots, corn, spinach, and beets did not trigger her uncomfortable symptoms, but that even *cooked* cabbage, broccoli, and Brussels sprouts caused her trouble. So, on Jennifer's personal food guide pyramid, we wrote lists of "Eat" and "Don't Eat" vegetables in the vegetable group. Raw vegetables and salad were at the top of her "Don't Eat" list.

Jennifer had also discovered from her journal that fruits eaten with the skin, such as grapes, cherries, and plums also contributed to her diarrhea, but citrus fruits, bananas, cantaloupes, mangos, and papayas were safe for her to eat. On her personal food guide pyramid, she wrote her lists of "Eat" and "Don't Eat" fruits in the fruit group. Because Jennifer's selection of fruits and vegetables was somewhat limited, I was concerned that she might not get sufficient fiber in her diet. Therefore I recommended that she supplement her diet with psyllium or another bulk-forming agent, which can be found at health food stores, drugstores, and even some supermarkets.

Jennifer's journal analysis also unveiled the fact that during times when diarrhea was a particular problem for her, such as during times of unusual stress, whole grain breads and cereals—especially those with bran—and brown rice made her diarrhea worse. I recommended that she avoid these grain products whenever she has diarrhea until the diarrhea goes away. Jennifer had found that oatmeal, potatoes, and white rice, white bread, and plain pasta did not aggravate her diarrhea. She noted this on her food guide pyramid in the grains section.

Jennifer had not detected any problems with dairy products when she examined her journal entries, so she left the milk group section of her pyramid the same as the regular food group pyramid.

In the meat/poultry/fish/dried beans/eggs/nuts section of Jennifer's personal food guide pyramid, she noted that cooked dried beans aggravated her gas and bloating, so she listed them under the "Don't Eat" column.

At the bottom of Jennifer's food guide pyramid, she added some notes: "Avoid coffee, tea, hot chocolate, and alcohol when you have diarrhea." Her journal indicated that these, too, seemed to make her diarrhea worse.

Jennifer now had a personalized version of the food guide pyramid that she had tailored to her specific reactions to various foods. I encouraged her to refer to it often when planning and preparing meals so that she would get a well-rounded diet of foods that wouldn't trigger her gastrointestinal symptoms.

Here are examples of three nutritious meals Jennifer could eat following her personal food guide pyramid:

BREAKFAST
- Milk, nonfat, 1 cup
- Oatmeal, 1 cup
- Banana, 1 cup, sliced over oatmeal
- White toast, 2 slices
- Diet margarine, 2 teaspoons
- Orange juice, 8 ounces

LUNCH
- Turkey, 3 ounces, sliced
- White bread, 2 slices
- Low-fat mozzarella cheese, 1 ounce
- Nonfat mayonnaise, 1 tablespoon
- Cantaloupe, 1 cup

DINNER

- Dinner roll, 1 small
- Diet margarine, 1 teaspoon
- Broiled swordfish steak, 3 ounces
- Mixed vegetable medley (green beans, carrots, and corn), ½ cup
- Baked potato, ½ medium
- Low-fat yogurt, ½ cup to top potato
- Mango, ripe, ½

Personal Food Guide Pyramid: IBS

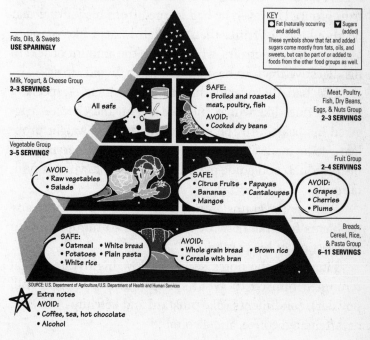

KEY
◯ Fat (naturally occurring and added)   ▼ Sugars (added)

These symbols show that fat and added sugars come mostly from fats, oils, and sweets, but can be part of or added to foods from the other food groups as well.

Fats, Oils, & Sweets
USE SPARINGLY

Milk, Yogurt, & Cheese Group
2–3 SERVINGS

All safe

Meat, Poultry, Fish, Dry Beans, Eggs, & Nuts Group
2–3 SERVINGS

SAFE:
- Broiled and roasted meat, poultry, fish

AVOID:
- Cooked dry beans

Vegetable Group
3–5 SERVINGS

AVOID:
- Raw vegetables
- Salads

Fruit Group
2–4 SERVINGS

SAFE:
- Citrus Fruits   • Papayas
- Bananas   • Cantaloupes
- Mangos

AVOID:
- Grapes
- Cherries
- Plums

SAFE:
- Oatmeal   • White bread
- Potatoes   • Plain pasta
- White rice

AVOID:
- Whole grain bread   • Brown rice
- Cereals with bran

Breads, Cereal, Rice, & Pasta Group
6–11 SERVINGS

SOURCE: U.S. Department of Agriculture/U.S. Department of Health and Human Services

✦ **Extra notes**
AVOID:
- Coffee, tea, hot chocolate
- Alcohol

Another patient, Hal, who suffered from heartburn, also created his own food guide pyramid using his food journal. Hal was overweight and had been instructed to lose weight by reducing his intake of fat and calories, so he wrote "AVOID" in big letters next to the top section of the pyramid: fats, oils and butters.

Next to the meat/poultry/fish/dried beans/eggs/nuts (2–3 servings) layer, Hal wrote "avoid fatty or fried meats" and "eat more broiled chicken and fish." Because Hal needed to increase his intake of fresh vegetables, he noted: "Be sure to eat 3–5 servings a day, but prepare them without added butter, oil, or bacon fat."

Similarly, he encouraged himself to eat two to four servings of fruits by writing, "Have fruit for dessert" next to the fruit group. However, he had learned from his journal that he should avoid fruits that are high in acid like oranges, lemons, and grapefruits, which add to the amount of acid in his digestive tract, so he made a note to "avoid citrus."

Hal had discovered that dairy products—especially high-fat ones like whole milk, ice cream, and cheese—triggered his heartburn (plus contributed to his weight problem), so he made a note in the milk group (2–3 servings) of his personal food guide pyramid that said, "low-fat or nonfat only."

Because the grains group had not seemed to cause any problems for Hal, he wrote, "Eat these to fill up" next to this section of his pyramid.

Finally, in the notes section below his pyramid, Hal reminded himself to avoid spices (like pepper and chili powder), condiments (like mustard and ketchup), caffeine, decaffeinated coffee, and alcohol.

FRIDGE ART

When my patients are getting used to the idea of watching what they eat, many have found it helpful to post a copy of their personal food guide pyramid on their refrigerator door. It reminds them to keep their day's food intake in proper balance while avoiding the particular foods proven to aggravate their gastrointestinal symptoms. You might also want to slip a copy into your wallet or purse for when you're shopping or eating out.

Then Hal posted his personal food guide pyramid on his refrigerator door as a reminder to eat a balanced array of foods and avoid those foods that cause his heartburn to flare up. Here are examples of three nutritious meals Hal could eat following his personal food guide pyramid:

BREAKFAST
- Milk, nonfat, 1 cup
- 100% bran cereal, 1 cup
- Fresh blackberries or strawberries, 1 cup, sliced over cereal
- Whole-wheat toast, 2 slices
- Apple butter, 2 tablespoons (on toast)
- Apple juice, 8 ounces

LUNCH
- Tuna salad made with:
    Tuna fish, 3 ounces, canned in water
    Celery, 1 stalk, chopped
    Lettuce, romaine, two leaves

Multigrain bread, 2 slices
Nonfat mayonnaise, 2 tablespoons
- Cantaloupe, 1 cup

DINNER
- Dinner roll, 1 small
- Diet margarine, 1 teaspoon
- Grilled chicken, 3 ounces
- Broccoli, ½ cup
- Brown and wild rice, 1 cup
- Salad with vinaigrette, 1 cup
- Pear, ripe, sliced, with skin

Personal Food Guide Pyramid: Heartburn

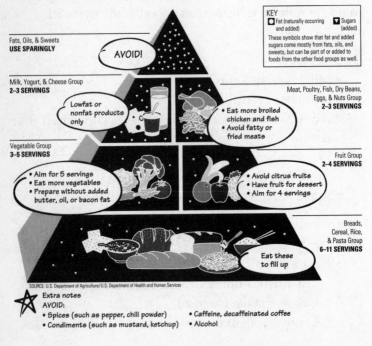

KEY
🔴 Fat (naturally occurring and added)   🔻 Sugars (added)
These symbols show that fat and added sugars come mostly from fats, oils, and sweets, but can be part of or added to foods from the other food groups as well.

Fats, Oils, & Sweets
USE SPARINGLY

AVOID!

Milk, Yogurt, & Cheese Group
2–3 SERVINGS

Lowfat or nonfat products only

Meat, Poultry, Fish, Dry Beans, Eggs, & Nuts Group
2–3 SERVINGS

- Eat more broiled chicken and fish
- Avoid fatty or fried meats

Vegetable Group
3–5 SERVINGS

- Aim for 5 servings
- Eat more vegetables
- Prepare without added butter, oil, or bacon fat

Fruit Group
2–4 SERVINGS

- Avoid citrus fruits
- Have fruit for dessert
- Aim for 4 servings

Breads, Cereal, Rice, & Pasta Group
6–11 SERVINGS

Eat these to fill up

SOURCE: U.S. Department of Agriculture/U.S. Department of Health and Human Services

Extra notes
AVOID:
- Spices (such as pepper, chili powder)
- Condiments (such as mustard, ketchup)
- Caffeine, decaffeinated coffee
- Alcohol

Ellen, another patient, suffered almost exclusively from gas and bloating. Here's how she constructed her personal food pyramid. Ellen started at the top of her pyramid and wrote "use sparingly" for fats, oils and butters. Ellen had noted when she went over her journal entries that she often experienced gas and bloating after eating milk or cheese. So, next to the milk, yogurt, and cheese group (2–3 servings), she wrote: "Eat only lactose-free dairy products, or use Lactaid. Yogurt okay to eat."

Next to the meat/poultry/fish/dried beans/eggs/nuts (2–3 servings) layer, Ellen wrote: "Avoid beans and nuts." Next to the vegetable group (3–5 servings), she wrote: "Don't eat cabbage, broccoli, cauliflower, Brussels sprouts, turnips, leeks, onions, or corn." Fruits hadn't seemed to give Ellen any problems, so she simply wrote "2–4 servings/day" next to the fruit section. Because she knew that breads contain lactose, which can cause gas and bloating, she wrote "Everything O.K. except bread" next to the breads, cereal, rice, and pasta group.

Here are examples of three nutritious meals Ellen could eat following her personal food guide pyramid:

BREAKFAST
- Lactose-free milk, nonfat, 1 cup
- French toast, 2 slices (made with 1 egg, ¼ cup lactose-free nonfat milk, and two slices whole-wheat bread)
- Fresh peaches, 1 cup, sliced, with skin

LUNCH
- Turkey sandwich made with:
  Rye bread, 2 slices

Sliced turkey, 3 ounces
Tomato, 3 slices
Lettuce, 1 leaf
- Cranberry juice, ³⁄₄ cup
- Frozen yogurt, ½ cup

DINNER

- Dinner roll, 1 small
- Grilled chicken, 3 ounces
- Spinach, ½ cup
- Stewed tomatoes, ½ cup
- Brown and wild rice, 1 cup
- Fruit salad, 1 cup

Personal Food Guide Pyramid: Gas and Bloating

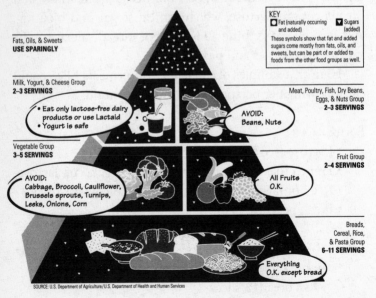

KEY
◻ Fat (naturally occurring and added) ▼ Sugars (added)
These symbols show that fat and added sugars come mostly from fats, oils, and sweets, but can be part of or added to foods from the other food groups as well.

Fats, Oils, & Sweets
USE SPARINGLY

Milk, Yogurt, & Cheese Group
2–3 SERVINGS
- Eat only lactose-free dairy products or use Lactaid
- Yogurt is safe

Meat, Poultry, Fish, Dry Beans, Eggs, & Nuts Group
2–3 SERVINGS
AVOID: Beans, Nuts

Vegetable Group
3–5 SERVINGS
AVOID: Cabbage, Broccoli, Cauliflower, Brussels sprouts, Turnips, Leeks, Onions, Corn

Fruit Group
2–4 SERVINGS
All Fruits O.K.

Breads, Cereal, Rice, & Pasta Group
6–11 SERVINGS
Everything O.K. except bread

SOURCE: U.S. Department of Agriculture/U.S. Department of Health and Human Services

Another patient, Ingrid, frequently suffered from constipation. After examining her journal, she, too, saw how she could create her own food pyramid. The areas of the basic food pyramid that Ingrid needed to make special notes on were the fruits; vegetables; bread, cereal, rice; and pasta sections. She needed to increase her intake of fruits, cooked vegetables, whole-grain breads and cereals, and liquids (fruit and vegetable juices and water). Here's an example of a day's menu for Ellen:

BREAKFAST
- Whole-grain cereal, 1 cup
- Blackberries, ½ cup
- Cantaloupe, 1 wedge
- Milk, nonfat, 1 cup
- Prune juice, ¾ cup

LUNCH
- Cooked zucchini and tomatoes, ½ cup each
- Mozzarella cheese, low-fat, 1 ounce
- Brown rice, 1 cup
- Orange juice, ¾ cup

DINNER
- Spaghetti with marinara sauce, 1 cup
- Italian breadsticks, 2
- Salad with Italian dressing, 1 cup
- Vanilla ice cream, low-fat, ½ cup
- Raspberries, ½ cup
- Grape juice, ¾ cup

Getting Started with Dietary Changes

Once you've created your own personal food guide pyramid, it's time to start implementing the dietary changes you've decided to make. As we discussed in chapter 2, it's important to make changes gradually, so as not to disrupt the status quo all at once. After reviewing patients' journals, I often help them list a menu of possible changes they could tackle, then ask them to select just one to try first. Because some people have more trouble making dietary changes than others do, some of my patients have made only minor changes while others are able to tolerate slightly bigger ones. Here are just a few of the smart "switches" my patients have decided to make as the very first step in their program for eliminating high-fat foods from their diet:

- Switch from whole milk to 2% to 1% (and eventually nonfat) milk. If you can't tolerate a complete switch all at once, try mixing whole milk with increasingly larger proportions of lowfat milk so that you have time to get used to the new taste.
- Switch from cheeseburgers to hamburgers and skip the fries. When you make your own hamburgers, buy the leanest ground beef.
- Substitute ground turkey for ground beef in home-made hamburgers.
- Start eating a piece of fruit for dessert instead of high-fat pastries or ice cream.
- Switch from ice cream to nonfat frozen yogurt for dessert.

- Switch from ordering pizza with "the works" to ordering veggie pizza.
- Switch from eating fat-laden croissants to whole-wheat dinner rolls or toast.

One of the best "first steps" patients can make isn't a dietary one, however. It's to begin adding physical exercise (such as a daily walk) to their routine. We'll discuss this all-important subject in detail in chapter 4.

I have found that for most people trying to eliminate an unhealthy food habit, such as drinking alcohol or coffee (both of which weaken the LES), slowing to a halt is usually more successful than going "cold turkey." If you're a five-cup-a-day coffee drinker and stop suddenly, you'll likely experience lethargy and withdrawal headaches. It's easier to cut back by one cup every few days or weeks. The idea is to make just one change at a time and to break up big changes into small incremental steps. It's much easier to take a series of small steps than to make giant leaps. Plus, small steps are key to effecting permanent change. Trying to change everything at once, on the other hand, is a guarantee of failure. Many of my patients have found it works best for them to make the easier changes first so they have a foundation for success and increased confidence to make the harder changes. Once you've successfully switched from whole milk to nonfat (skim) milk, for example, you'll be encouraged to try making another change, such as cutting down on caffeine. Over a period of time, your more healthful diet will unfold—one change at a time.

- *GO SLOW*
- To be most effective, any dietary changes you adopt should
- be gradual. Gradual changes are less disruptive, and there's a
- better chance that they'll become an integral part of your life.

Learn New Ways to Prepare Foods

The ways that you prepare foods can affect whether they contribute to your GI symptoms. For instance, people who have irritable bowel syndrome frequently have trouble when they eat raw vegetables, but experience no symptoms if the same vegetables have been cooked. In the same way, vegetables that have been fried or cooked in bacon fat or butter can worsen symptoms. Cooking rice or vegetables in low-fat chicken broth or vegetable broth instead of fat may make them not only tasty but also tolerable to your digestive tract.

Beth, the wife of Frank, one of my patients, was a stay-at-home mom who prided herself on the way she managed the family's household, coached soccer for her young boys and their teammates, and prepared wonderful gourmet meals every night. Unfortunately, Beth's idea of a gourmet meal was one prepared in the traditional French manner, with lots of cream and butter. She also deep-fried many foods to give them a crispy crust before covering them with a creamy sauce. Frank, my patient, loved his wife's cooking and often invited clients and coworkers home to taste her cuisine. When Frank came to me complaining of heartburn, he wanted me to give him a prescription for some sort of medicine to make his symptoms go away so he could continue to enjoy Beth's wonderful cooking. I'm afraid that I disappointed him when, instead, I prescribed that Beth enroll in a low-fat cooking class at our local adult school.

Frank balked at the idea, saying that he and his family wouldn't want her to change anything about her cooking methods because her meals were so delicious just the way they were. But, as his symptoms grew worse over time, he finally mentioned the idea to Beth. Eager to do anything she could to make Frank's heartburn go away, she signed up for the next available class. Soon she was cooking with low-sodium defatted chicken broth and a splash of wine instead of bacon drippings, oils, and butter—and she was learning techniques for bringing out the flavors of foods with fresh herbs instead of covering them up with heavy sauces. According to Frank, she had become an even better cook. As for Frank, he lost some weight and his heartburn improved—and he continues to invite guests over to sample Beth's cooking every chance he gets.

NEW WAYS TO COOK

To learn new ways to prepare your favorite foods, try taking healthful, low-fat cooking classes at your local community college, adult school, or gourmet food shop. Or check out the diet cookbook section of your bookstore or library for low-fat recipes. Foods prepared by steaming, roasting, broiling, grilling, or microwaving are lower in fat than those sautéed in butter or deep fried in oil. Try sautéing foods in low-sodium, defatted broth or use a non-stick cooking spray. Learn to use fresh herbs to add flavor without adding fat or sodium. (See Resources at the end of this book for recommended low-fat cookbooks.)

Making Healthy Food Choices When You Eat Out

If you're trying to cut down on fat and calories, you don't have to stop eating out. Making healthy food choices at restaurants isn't as difficult as you may think. There are foods you can eat on almost every menu. First, consider how the dish is cooked. Look for grilled chicken or fish instead of fried foods. Steamed vegetables are a good choice, but be sure to ask for them to be served without butter or other high-fat sauces. In Chinese restaurants, look for dishes with lots of vegetables, such as chicken chow mein. In Italian restaurants, look for pasta with marinara sauce. In Mexican restaurants, ask them to hold the sour cream and cheese, and order chicken, shrimp, or vegetable fajitas. Always keep portion sizes in mind, as many restaurants serve portions large enough for two people to share. If you don't choose to split your entrée with a dining partner, be sure to leave half on your plate or take it home in a doggy bag. With practice, you'll find that ordering a tasty healthful meal on the town is as easy as remembering to say, "Hold the pie."

NO PIZZA ON FRIDAY
Many people eat out of habit. If you automatically buy hot dogs at the ball game, buttered popcorn at the movies, or delivery pizza on Friday nights, focus on breaking those habits. Soon, you won't even miss them.

Dietary Do's and Don'ts

For People with Heartburn
If you suffer from heartburn or acid indigestion, you may find the following recommendations helpful:

- If you are overweight, eat fewer calories—especially fewer calories from fats—so that you lose weight.
- Eat smaller meals. Big meals take longer to digest and cause the stomach to produce more acid.
- Avoid drinks that contain caffeine—such as coffee, black tea, cola drinks, and hot chocolate. When it comes to coffee, even the decaffeinated kind can cause acid reflux. Use your food journal to carefully record whether it's coffee or coffee with cream that triggers your symptoms. Many of my patients have discovered that it's the steamed whole milk in their latte that's the culprit.
- If you can't give up your morning coffee, try drinking a big glass of water after it to dilute the coffee's effect. Gradually drink weaker and weaker coffee, and cut down on the number of cups you drink.
- Avoid mint-flavored foods, including after-dinner mints, mint teas, mint candies, and gums. Oil of peppermint relaxes the valve between the esophagus and the stomach (the LES), allowing acid to seep back up.
- Avoid chocolate, which, like peppermint, lowers the LES pressure and allows greater acid reflux.
- Try sucking on non-mint candies or lozenges that stimulate the flow of saliva, which can neutralize the acid in your esophagus. Salivation normally decreases at night, so many of my patients have found that popping a candy in their mouth eases nighttime heartburn.
- Avoid alcohol, another culprit that relaxes the valve between the esophagus and the stomach, and also stimulates the production of acid.

- Avoid cigarette smoking. Nicotine may irritate the lining of the throat and disrupt normal digestion.
- Many people who experience heartburn find relief when they avoid dairy products—especially high-fat ones like whole milk, ice cream, and cheeses.
- Avoid foods that are high in acid—such as oranges, lemons, grapefruits, and tomatoes (including ketchup), which add to the amount of acid in your digestive tract.
- Use your food journal to determine which spices and condiments—such as mustard, pepper, and hot sauce—contribute to your uncomfortable symptoms.
- Plan your evening meal so that you have three or four hours after eating before you lie down.

A SOUPÇON OF SAUCE

When eating out, learn to ask for sauces and salad dressings on the side. Then lightly dip the prongs of your fork into the sauce or dressing before you pick up a forkful of food. You'll get to taste the high-fat flavor without consuming too much of it.

For People with Gas or Bloating

If you experience excess gassiness, you may find it helpful to:

- Eliminate gas-forming foods—cabbage, broccoli, cauliflower, coleslaw, corn, beans, nuts, carbonated beverages—for a while. You may reintroduce them gradually once your gas symptoms have gone away. Use your food journal to help figure out which foods contribute to excess gas in your particular case.

- Decrease your chance of swallowing air by avoiding chewing gum, hard candy, cigarettes, and carbonated beverages.
- Avoid drinking lots of liquids with your meals.
- Eat slowly and chew your food thoroughly.

For People with Constipation

The following is a list of basic guidelines to facilitate a healthy bowel routine:

- Increase fiber and roughage in your diet by including foods such as fruits, cooked vegetables, whole-grain breads and cereals, and bran. (If you have diarrhea, however, you should exclude fiber from your diet until the diarrhea goes away.) Increase the fiber in your diet gradually, since adding too much fiber too rapidly will cause gas pains. Your doctor may recommend that you take a fiber supplement, such as Metamucil, which contains psyllium. Do not, however, get into the habit of using laxatives unless your doctor recommends them. You could become dependent on them.
- Eat at regular hours. Eat three meals daily. Skipping meals and then eating on an empty stomach can wreak havoc with your digestive system and aggravate uncomfortable symptoms.
- Chew food slowly and thoroughly.
- Decrease your chance of swallowing air by avoiding chewing gum, hard candy, and carbonated beverages.
- Drink six to eight cups of liquid daily, including fruit and vegetable juices and water. Coffee doesn't count, since it acts as a diuretic.

- Maintain a regular program of physical exercise and activity.
- Avoid delaying the urge to have a bowel movement. Avoid straining; try to relax and take your time.
- Establish a routine time and place for having a bowel movement. Many people find that right after breakfast is a good time; and most people are more comfortable doing this at home, perhaps while reading the daily newspaper.

For People with Diarrhea

- Use your food journal to detect foods (such as dairy products, chocolate, eggs, or wheat products) that trigger your diarrhea. Sometimes diarrhea is caused by a food intolerance.
- Similarly, use your journal to determine whether stress triggers your diarrhea.
- Remember that you can become dehydrated when you have persistent diarrhea, so be sure to rehydrate with plenty of water. You probably don't need the expensive "sports drinks" to refuel if you drink at least six to eight glasses of water daily.

Throughout this chapter, I've given you suggestions for foods to look for in your journal that may be causing your particular digestive symptoms. Because fat is often the most troublesome component in my patients' diets, I have recommended ways to limit your fat intake—from recognizing high-fat foods to cutting portions down to size, to learning low-fat cooking methods. These techniques have helped many of my patients lower their consumption of fat and lose some weight. But it's important to note that food is only one part of a successful regimen for weight loss—exercise is needed to complete the program. We'll discuss how exercise can complement your healthful diet in the next chapter.

4

Get Moving:
One Prescription for Many GI Conditions

....

WHAT if I could give you a single prescription that could have a positive impact not only on many of your digestive symptoms but also on several other aspects of your life? Believe it or not, *regular physical activity* is just that prescription—but it's often the hardest prescription to convince my patients to begin to take.

I've heard all the excuses: "I never liked to exercise"; "I don't have the time"; "I just can't stick with an exercise program." In this chapter, I hope to show you that exercise doesn't have to be a bitter pill to swallow. In fact, it should be enjoyable. By following the suggestions I make, you can gradually and painlessly incorporate a healthful dose of physical activity into your daily routine.

Where Did All the Exercise Go?

First, it's important to understand why we are exercising less. As machines and computers made our daily lives easier, we humans have lost many of our reasons to exercise. We no longer need to chase wild game or till the soil before we can eat. Instead, our hunting and gathering takes place as we stroll the aisles of the supermarket. Once we've brought home the bacon, we rarely spend much energy in food preparation. Even chores such as kneading bread, chopping vegetables, opening cans, and washing dishes—which used to get people moving a little—have been taken over by machines.

FIND A FUN EXERCISE

For many of my patients, the first thing I have to convince them to do is to change their *attitude* about exercise. While some people enjoy active sports and exercise, others insist they hate changing into sportswear and getting sweaty. For some, the mere notion of physical activity conjures up reminiscences of stern high school gym teachers who forced them to run extra laps around the baseball field as punishment for being late for class. The key is to discover that there are many different ways of getting exercise—and to find a form of exercise that you will *enjoy* so that you will stick with it.

Regular Exercise Helps Relieve GI Distress and More

Although we don't understand exactly *how* exercise works to alleviate symptoms such as gas and bloating, the observation that this occurs had been made many times. I think that most doctors would agree that regular exercise helps promote normal intestinal function, which in turn helps pass gas, reduces bloating and cramping, and results in more regular bowel habits. Many of my patients have told me that their bowel function improved once they started a regular exercise program. It may be that exercise stimulates the production of chemicals called *endorphins* in the nervous system and that these chemicals help regulate bowel function. Or, it may be that exercise simply increases intestinal motility on a physical rather than a chemical level. Motility allows us to pass small amounts of gas, reducing the sensations of bloating, belching, distention, and fullness.

NO JUMPING!

If you have heartburn, be aware that the kinds of exercise in which you jump up and down or bounce a lot—such as jogging, aerobic dancing, or using a stair-stepping machine— will stimulate your condition. I recommend to patients who have heartburn that they try non-jarring types of low-impact exercise, such as swimming or walking, to encourage healthy bowel motility and relieve stress and anxiety.

Exercise helps relieve stress and depression, both of which compromise gastrointestinal health in those with sensitive digestive systems. Because it helps relieve stress, exercise may decrease the pain associated with ulcers and the symptoms of irritable bowel syndrome. In addition to helping alleviate digestive symptoms, there are other potential physical and mental benefits of regular exercise. Exercise improves physical stamina and lessens fatigue. It lowers your blood pressure and cholesterol and triglyceride levels, which, in turn, lessens your risk of having a heart attack or developing coronary artery disease. Regular exercise increases your mobility and flexibility, tones flabby muscles, and improves your posture. Weight-bearing forms of exercise—like walking or jogging—can help keep your bones strong. And that's not all—exercise reduces body fat and improves your appearance, energy level, and overall self-image. My experience has been that when my patients improve their outlook and attitude through exercise, they become more motivated to make other beneficial changes.

You don't necessarily have to join an expensive gym or buy fancy equipment to incorporate a moderate amount of exercise into your daily routine—walking your dog in the evening or taking a walk around the parking lot at work during your lunch break, dancing, swimming laps, biking, and similar types of low-impact activities qualify as exercise as long as you keep up the movement without interruption for at least thirty minutes. But if your walks involve stopping every few minutes for your dog to sniff the bushes or for you to window-shop, or if your swimming sessions are interrupted with periods of floating or holding on to the side of the pool, they don't count as true workouts. Activities like gardening, golf, tennis, and actively playing with children may get you moving a little, but they don't qualify as a daily workout because they don't involve continuous movement.

If you're trying to lose weight, don't assume that exercise gives you license to eat whatever you want. I remember a cooperative and well-meaning patient who finally agreed to start exercising. He learned to enjoy bicycle riding and soon was biking ten miles a day. Each month he came to see me, he reported that his gastrointestinal symptoms had improved, but I noted a gradual increase in his weight in spite of his increased exercise. After questioning him, I found out that, though in the beginning he was riding in the mornings, he had moved his workouts to the evenings as he increased his mileage so he'd have time to ride without worrying about being late for work.

ACCENTUATE THE POSITIVE

Many of my patients who had several behaviors to change, such as stopping smoking, avoiding alcohol, cutting down on fats and spices in their diet, and adding exercise to their routine, have found that it's easier at first to *add* a *positive* behavior than it is to *discontinue* a *negative* one. Once you've successfully added a thirty-minute walk to your daily routine, you'll be encouraged to make other healthful changes, such as eliminating drinking wine with your evening meal.

By riding in the evenings, right after work, he was ravenously hungry when he finally got around to having dinner—his large evening meals often stretched to eleven o'clock. Because he was exercising so much, he didn't worry about how much food he was consuming, and his caloric intake rose.

He was not the only patient I've observed who thought that heavy exercise in the evenings gave him license to eat a heavy evening meal. Many patients are so tired after their workouts that not only do they feel they need to eat heavily but they feel they "need" to drink alcohol for greater relaxation. This regimen just adds more calories and more problems.

Stepping Up

As we discussed in chapter 2, it's important to make lifestyle changes gradually, one step at a time. Radical changes rarely stick, because they cause too much disruption in your life. And with exercise, too much too soon can lead to injuries.

TWICE AS LIKELY TO QUIT

According to a recent study led by Dr. Bess Marcus of Brown University School of Medicine, if you're trying to kick the smoking habit, adding regular exercise to the attempt is likely to boost your chances for success. In this study, published in the Annals of Internal Medicine, all 281 of the participants were women smokers who, prior to the study, were not exercising regularly. The women were divided into two groups: one group followed a twelve-week smoking-cessation program, while the other group followed the smoking-cessation program plus a three-times-weekly exercise regimen. The researchers found that the exercisers were twice as likely to quit smoking and to remain smoke-free for a year than the group that was not exercising. The exercisers also tended to gain less weight during the study than the inactive group. Besides minimizing weight gain, exercise can ease the stress, depression, and anxiety that go along with quitting smoking.

If you're just beginning an exercise program, the key is to start slowly and to work up to a half hour nearly every day. I often suggest that my patients begin with ten minutes a day and add ten minutes every other day or so—

depending on the individual—until they are exercising at least thirty minutes a day. While it's generally believed that thirty *consecutive* minutes of aerobic exercise provide the greatest benefit, recent studies have shown that it's acceptable to grab ten or fifteen exercise minutes here and there throughout the day, as long as the day's cumulative exercise time adds up to thirty minutes.

You Know Best What Will Work for You

To get started incorporating more physical activity into your daily routine, think about what's available to you and what you like to do. Do you have access to gym equipment or a community swimming pool? What kinds of active sports do you enjoy or have enjoyed in the past?

PICK AN EXERCISE—NOT JUST ANY EXERCISE

To help you pick a few types of exercise that suit you best, start by listing all the kinds of exercise or sports that you've enjoyed in the past—as well as any new sports or activities that you've always wanted to try. Walking, jogging, swimming laps, bicycling or riding an exercise bike, cross-country skiing (on skis or a skiing machine), rowing, in-line skating, aerobic dance, water aerobics, jumping rope, and stair climbing (either on a stair-step machine or on real stairs) are all good examples of aerobic activities. Tennis, soccer, racquetball, volleyball, basketball, golfing (using a hand cart or carrying your own clubs), ballroom dancing, gardening, lawn mowing (using a mower you push), raking leaves, washing and waxing your car, or pushing a stroller can be used to supplement your aerobic exercise regimen.

Everyone's different. So, before you fork over a hefty annual membership fee at a fitness center, ask yourself if you'll enjoy working out in front of people or if you're the type of person who prefers to exercise alone. For some people, exercise is a form of socializing and meeting new people, or they may need a class to stay motivated, but for others, especially those who prefer walking, swimming laps, or riding a stationary bike, exercise means a welcome time of solitude during which they get some of their best ideas. Still other people like to engage in recreational sports, such as tennis, golf, racquetball, or hiking for part of their exercise program.

What types of exercise will you really *do?* One of my patients who knew that she couldn't break herself of her evening television habit found that a treadmill positioned right in front of the TV was the best way to get herself moving. If you decide to try this route, you may want to rent a treadmill before buying one—or perhaps look for a used one in the classified advertisements in your local newspaper. Or consider trying out a similar piece of equipment at a health club or gym for a month or two—using a guest pass or a temporary membership—to see if it can hold your interest. Exercise equipment is expensive, and too many people end up using treadmills, stationary bicycles, rowing machines, or cross-country skiing machines for little more than hat racks and clothes trees after a few months. Finding a form of exercise that's best for you is often a trial-and-error process.

Anything we do can be overdone or done improperly to our detriment, even though it is done with the best intentions. For example, I remember one thirty-three-year-old businessman who became an avid bodybuilder when he was in his twenties. He had irritable bowel syndrome and managed relatively well with his gas, bloating, diarrhea alternating with constipation, and abdominal cramping throughout his teenage years and early twenties. After several years of weight lifting, however, he developed mild heartburn. It was mild at first, but progressively increased in severity and was associated with a bitter taste in his mouth. His symptoms went untreated, and eventually he experienced episodes of sudden pain in the middle of his chest, often associated with a feeling that he needed to belch in order to get relief from his discomfort. Eventually, he began experiencing a sensation of pressure in his chest, heartburn that became progressively more severe, and worse episodes of chest pain. His physicians determined that his weight lifting, which had become a passion, had weakened the muscles in his diaphragm where the stomach and esophagus come together. A previous hiatal hernia—caused when the upper portion of the stomach lifts above the diaphragm—had been made worse by his weight lifting, and now acid was able to flow freely from his stomach into his esophagus. He was advised to reduce his weight lifting to a point where he did not have to grunt (this is called a Valsalva maneuver) when he lifted weights. I recommended he substitute aerobic exercise for weight lifting to better control his other abdominal symptoms, and told him to avoid gas-producing foods. As he reduced the amount of weight lifting he was doing, his symptoms of heartburn, chest pain and pressure became less frequent and severe. By making dietary changes and beginning a program of regular aerobic exercise (which in his case consisted of long-distance bicycle riding), his lower abdominal symptoms came under control.

Walking GI Distress Right Out of Your Life

Dozens of my patients with GI problems, especially those with heartburn, have found that running and other forms of high-impact exercise that cause a lot of jostling of the body induce symptoms. For that reason, I recommend brisk walking, swimming, or riding a bicycle over jogging or running for most of my patients. In fact, I consider walking to be one of the best forms of exercise—especially for people who aren't used to working out. It's as easy as putting one foot in front of the other! Other than good shoes, you don't need special equipment, clothing, or facilities to walk. You can walk in the city or in the country, alone or with company, with or without a dog (as long as Fido doesn't slow you down). By dressing appropriately, you can walk in almost any weather. You can even walk indoors at a shopping mall in bad weather, although it's important that you don't slow down to window-shop. Some malls welcome walkers before regular shopping hours. If business causes you to travel a lot, you can always ask the hotel desk clerk for safe walking course suggestions in an unfamiliar town. Walking is a wonderful way to explore a new place, since you'll catch many sights you'd miss by driving.

If you live in a climate where weather often prevents you from walking outside, you may want to consider getting a treadmill so you can walk in your home virtually any time of any day.

- ***TALK YES, SING NO***
- To find out whether you're exercising at the right pace, use this rule: you should be able to carry on a conversation with a training partner. If you're too winded to complete a sentence, you're going too fast. On the other hand, if you can sing a tune while you're working out, you should probably pick up the pace.

Depending on your personal style, you can time your walks, setting a thirty- or forty-five-minute walk as your goal each day, or you can get a pedometer and keep track of the number of miles you've walked. One of my patients tacked up a map of the country on her bulletin board, logged her mileage, and pretended she was traveling on a long road trip. Each week, she'd add up the miles she'd covered, calculate with the map which city she was in, and mark the map with a pin. If you think this kind of mind trip might inspire you to keep walking, try it.

There are both pros and cons to walking with a partner. For some of my patients, having the partner waiting outside helped motivate them to walk even on days when they felt like skipping their workout. But the purpose of your walk can be defeated if your partner slows you down. Too often, you get involved in conversation and forget to keep up the pace. I usually suggest that my patients who choose to walk with someone else do so quietly.

In most cases, I think walking solo is best. You can concentrate on keeping your pace brisk and let your lungs fill with oxygen and your thoughts wander. One of my patients, a forty-eight-year-old mystery novelist, claims that she often gets ideas for plot and character development during her afternoon walks.

When my patients are beginning a walking program, I give them the following tips to ensure a healthy start, as well as to get the most benefit from their walks:

- Get your doctor's go-ahead before you begin. This is important for everyone, and is especially critical if you're overweight or unaccustomed to physical activity or if you have a chronic health problem such as heart disease, diabetes, asthma, or a lung, joint, or muscular disorder.
- Do some light leg-muscle stretches before your walk, but save the heavy stretching for immediately afterward, while your muscles are warm.
- Each walking session should begin with a warm-up period, during which you gradually increase the pace of your walk, to prevent muscle strain, and end with a cool-down period to ease your body's transition back to a resting state.
- The middle, or main part of your walk should be brisk enough so that you can feel you're working harder. Walk quickly enough to deepen your breathing comfortably and increase your heart rate—but not so fast that you couldn't carry on a conversation or that you find yourself panting for breath.
- Bend your arms from the elbow at a right angle and swing them naturally with each step.
- Don't use hand weights while walking. They could

increase your blood pressure and contribute to joint problems.

- Invest in good walking shoes and athletic socks. When shopping for shoes, consider whether you'll be doing more walking on flat pavement or off the road, such as along the beach or in the woods, because rougher terrain requires a thicker sole. Finally, to avoid injury, replace your shoes before they look worn out.

- Don't compare yourself with others. If other walkers pass you by, that's okay as long as you're getting a good workout. Over time, you can gradually increase your activity intensity.

- Don't forget to reward yourself for every step of progress. If you're a beginner, even once around the block can be an accomplishment worthy of a reward. Just make sure that you celebrate with a healthful reward—a subscription to a health magazine, a new workout outfit, a warm bath, a movie, or a favorite author's newest book—but not a trip to the bakery for doughnuts!

SET YOUR TIMER

To be sure you walk for at least thirty minutes, it's helpful to carry a timer with you. If you're walking the same route every day, you'll soon learn how far you can go in thirty minutes, but if you sometimes take different paths, the timer can help you make sure you've walked long enough. No matter where you are (even if you're in an unfamiliar city), if you're planning to walk for thirty minutes, you can set the timer for fifteen minutes and, when the buzzer goes off, you'll know it's time to turn around and head back.

Common Sense Walking Guidelines

Whenever you go walking, it's important to use common sense and be aware of your surroundings. Before I send my patients out walking for the first time, I offer them the following tips to ensure their safety:

- Always walk facing traffic.
- Walk on sidewalks where possible, or stay close to the side of the road.
- Wear reflective clothing and carry a flashlight if you're walking after dark.
- Carry identification, but leave expensive jewelry and watches at home. Walk with a companion whenever possible, especially in a deserted area.
- If you do walk alone, let someone know you're going walking, your route, and when you expect to return.
- Don't use headphones if you're walking alone in an unfamiliar area, exercising at night, or in heavy traffic.
- Apply sunscreen if you'll be walking during the day to avoid sunburn.

Aerobic Exercise Is the Key

It's important to choose a type of exercise for your regular workouts that's aerobic. Aerobic exercise is the kind that gets your heart rate up and keeps you moving for an extended period of time (thirty minutes or more). Walking, jogging, and swimming laps are examples of aerobic exercise. I remember one patient who was thirty pounds overweight who came to me complaining of heartburn and indigestion. His heartburn was probably aggravated by his weight. Heavy people tend to have a greater reflux of acid from the stomach up into the esophagus from swallowing. And people who have heartburn usually have weakening of the *lower esophageal sphincter;* the band of muscle that separates the esophagus from the stomach and prevents acid from moving from the stomach up into the swallowing tube.

DO TREAD ON ME

One of my patients, a business executive with irritable bowel syndrome, started an outdoor walking program. He was amazed at how much better he felt when he exercised. But business commitments often caused him to work late, and he sometimes had to forfeit his after-work walks. His solution was to buy a treadmill as a "reward" for succeeding with his walking regimen and put it in his office so he could steal a half hour or more during each day to walk away his gas, bloating, constipation, and stress. I now recommend that other patients try to place treadmills in their workplaces. Working out on a treadmill during your business day doesn't even require you to change clothes or shoes or to shower afterward. For the purposes of improving digestive health, it's not necessary that you exercise so hard that you sweat. If you can't afford to buy your own treadmill for your office, or if your work space isn't big enough to accommodate a large piece of exercise equipment, consider asking your company to provide a treadmill for the employees' lounge.

I asked him if he got any exercise. "Sure, Doc," he said, "I get plenty of exercise. I play golf every Saturday morning, and sometimes my wife, Dolores, and I play doubles tennis with another couple on Sundays at the club. I bowl on Thursday nights, too—we're in a league. And I lift weights at the gym. Yeah, I'm a pretty active guy."

I hated to burst his bubble, but I explained to him that he wasn't getting much *aerobic* exercise. I recommended that he start swimming for exercise each and every day, and that he stop lifting weights. I also advised him to avoid peppermint, chocolate, and spicy foods, spices (such as pepper), and condiments (such as mustard, ketchup, and hot sauce) that promote heartburn symptoms. I also recommended that he avoid wearing tight clothing and that he not recline within three hours after eating, because these things aggravate the symptoms of heartburn and indigestion. I advised him to start losing weight and to avoid large meals, which actually promote acid reflux.

THINNESS IS NOT THE GOAL

Exercise doesn't have to make you thin to do you a lot of good. While many people experience a slow, steady weight loss once they start an exercise program, your gastrointestinal health can improve from regular aerobic exercise, regardless of whether or not you lose weight. Too often people consider the big payoff from exercise to be cosmetic. They jog or lift weights to sculpt thin, beautiful bodies. But for many people, especially as they age, exercise can provide many benefits—including cardiovascular and digestive health—even if they are unable to lose all the weight they'd like to. I have many patients who, while still carrying some excess pounds, have dramatically improved their overall physical and mental health by undertaking a regular exercise program, such as daily walking.

I warned him that patients who fail to follow these recommendations—or whose symptoms do not respond to these simple strategies—may need to take acid-reducing medicines called proton-pump inhibitors. (We'll discuss these medications in chapter 6.)

At his next appointment six months later, he was beaming. "Doc, you were right about that swimming stuff. I've been swimming fifty laps at the YMCA pool every morning before breakfast, and I feel great! I've lost eight pounds and I sleep better at night. I've hardly needed to take any medicine for my stomach, either. You're a genius!"

A problem can crop up if people have overly optimistic expectations that their bodies will become thin and svelte because of their exercising. If they decide exercise hasn't done what they wanted it to do, they may become discouraged and give up exercising altogether. To avoid this pitfall, remind yourself of how much better you feel by keeping up your exercise habit, and refer to your journal to verify this cause-and-effect relationship. And, if weight loss is one of your goals, supplement your exercise program with a calorie-restricted diet to trim pounds.

Making Time for Exercise

Finding the time to exercise is often as much of a challenge as finding the right type of workout. I encourage my patients to start by thinking about which times of the day they're more likely to exercise. If you're a night person rather than a morning person, it's unlikely that you'll stick too long with a plan to get up an hour earlier every morning to go jogging. If you do like to get up early, however, you may prefer to work out first thing in the morning, shower afterward, and get on with your working day. Many of my patients who like to swim find they enjoy starting the day with laps in the pool. Other people seem to do better by unwinding with their exercise sessions after work.

ON THE ROAD

Traveling is no excuse for missing your regular workouts. Be sure your exercise gear and athletic shoes are the first items you pack. I suggest to all my patients who travel a lot for business or pleasure that before they make their hotel reservations, they find out about the kinds of exercise facilities the hotel has to offer. Look for both indoor and outdoor exercise options, so you won't be caught without an exercise option if the weather turns bad. Does the hotel have an indoor swimming pool? a treadmill?

When the weather permits, walking or jogging in a new or foreign city at dawn or dusk can provide a wonderful way to see the sights and get to know the city up close. You'll see the local shopkeepers going about their daily business, smell the flowers and bakeries, and hear the children playing— details you're likely to miss from a tour bus or taxicab.

There may also be biological reasons why one time of the day may be better than another for you to exercise. Because exercise stimulates the release of calming chemicals called *endorphins,* many people find that working out at the beginning of the day gets the day off to a pleasant, stress-reduced start, which in turn may lessen acid secretion and reduce the symptoms of heartburn or indigestion. Other patients obtain the optimal benefits of exercise by planning their workouts for the time when a break in their daily routine is most welcome. A brisk walk at midday stimulates intestinal motility, provides the calming effects of endorphin release, and allows you to return to work refreshed and invigorated for the second half of the day. Those people who have trouble unwinding after work without the help of alcohol may find that exercising at the end of the day will help them relax and lessen their dependence on alcohol as a tranquilizer. Plus, once they're able to start avoiding alcohol, they'll find that their heartburn and indigestion improve, because alcohol causes increased acid release.

Let me describe one patient's journey to find relief through exercise. This fifty-two-year-old businessman, living in a large metropolitan city, led a sedentary life. His day usually consisted of rising around 7:00 A.M., gulping down a glass of orange juice and a cup of coffee, rushing to work, sitting at his desk throughout the morning, sitting through a business lunch (often with a drink before and during lunch), followed by an afternoon spent sitting at his desk talking on the telephone—all the while doing very little in the form of physical movement. His workday extended into the early evening and he usually arrived home after 7:30 P.M. When he got home, he unwound with another cocktail. His dinner was the largest meal of his day. He preferred heavily spiced foods, which he consumed in large amounts. He generally had another drink after dinner, which relaxed him enough to go to bed early. Over many years, this lifestyle had resulted in his becoming more than forty pounds overweight.

After many months of nagging, his wife convinced him he should have a physical examination—which he hadn't done in more than a decade. When he came to see me, he was not only obese and complaining of indigestion and heartburn, but he also had high blood pressure and signs of an abnormal liver. Because of those abnormal liver tests, I ordered a liver biopsy, which, fortunately, revealed the earliest signs of alcoholic liver disease (called "fatty liver"), a totally reversible form of liver disease.

The diagnosis of a liver problem was frightening enough to the patient that it caused him to want to change his lifestyle. He stopped drinking alcohol, and switched to a high-protein, low-fat diet.

I encouraged him to begin exercising regularly, but he really disliked any form of physical activity. Throughout his life, he had never received any form of gratification from sports. When he was a child, the other kids ridiculed him because he was so unskilled in most sporting activities. However, with his children, his wife, and me, his physician, encouraging him, he joined a health club and began using a stair-climbing machine each morning. He gradually increased his activity on the machine until he was actually stepping for thirty consecutive minutes each morning. However, he found that his heartburn, which had greatly improved with his lifestyle changes, worsened as he increased his exercise activity. He became friendly with a trainer at his gym, who suggested that he try some other form of exercise. He began swimming laps, and after the first two weeks found it relaxing and enjoyable. He gradually increased the number of laps each day, and he soon observed that his indigestion and heartburn had disappeared. His weight loss increased, and he felt generally good.

Around that time, though, as his workload increased in his job, he found that each morning he was spending less and less time in the pool. He began experiencing increasing anxiety over the amount of work that was awaiting him in his office. Over a period of a few weeks, he found that, in spite of exercise and weight loss, he was again experiencing indigestion. He began exercising less as his anxiety about "missing" work increased. This became such a problem that he gave up morning exercise altogether—and of course found that many of his symptoms recurred.

SATURDAYS & SUNDAYS COUNT, TOO

Whatever time for exercise seems best for you, establish a schedule for when and where you're planning to work out all week. Post it in your kitchen or bathroom, or write it on your desk calendar—where you'll be sure to see it every day. If you just intend to work out whenever you find some spare time, you'll end up exercising infrequently. Also, make a separate plan for weekends to make sure you exercise on Saturdays and Sundays. For example, if your weekend activities include driving to the shore, pack your athletic shoes and plan to stop for a brisk walk on the beach. If you plan to have a picnic in the park with your family, ride bikes and pack a softball for some athletic fun. If you miss a planned exercise session, cross it off on your calendar and write in the activity you did to replace it.

At the suggestion of a friend, he attempted midday exercise followed by a small lunch. A brisk walk at noon gradually gave way to longer and longer periods of walking, followed by a relatively healthy high-protein, low-fat lunch, often consisting of fruit, cottage cheese, yogurt, and sometimes a turkey sandwich with nonfat milk. Midday exercise seemed to greatly reduce the anxiety he had experienced in the morning. The endorphin release he experienced from the exercise provided a tranquilizing effect, and over a period of twelve months he lost the forty pounds he had gained over the prior decade. At the end of that period, he was symptom-free, thin, and a much happier man.

Many of my patients have complained that they find it really hard to get started and to stick strictly to an exercise program because time is their obstacle. Having to work late at the office or pick up the children at day care can interfere with regular attendance at scheduled aerobics classes or fitness centers that are open only during certain hours. That's why I recommend that they plan backup exercise options for those days when they can't fit their regular exercise into the schedule. Any kind of activity is better than none—a brisk walk around the neighborhood, shooting baskets in the driveway with the kids, or even housework counts. One woman I know relies on exercise videos. She enjoys keeping up with the latest fitness craze—Tae Bo, kick-boxing, etc.—and keeps herself interested by alternating tapes. She doesn't have to worry that her schedule will preclude exercise—the tapes are ready to pop into the VCR at her convenience.

THE LONG HAUL

Start slow—don't overdo it when beginning an exercise program. The resulting aches and pains only discourage further exercise. So resist the urge to push yourself too hard and too soon. Instead, take it easy and gradually build up to more advanced levels. As the weeks go by, slowly increase the time that you stay active. By beginning slowly, you'll give your muscles, tendons, and bones a chance to adjust to the new workload and you'll reduce your chance of injury. Remember, you're in this for the long haul.

Staying Motivated

Once you've started exercising, the next challenge is to avoid becoming an exercise dropout when your enthusiasm wanes. Many of the principles you learned in chapter 2 can help. To provide a visual reminder of your success, you may want to post a calendar on your refrigerator door or bathroom mirror and check off each day you exercise. When you slip off your intended program, don't beat yourself up. Forgive yourself when you lapse. Try to figure out why the lapse happened and how you can avoid it next time. If you just can't seem to get up early to go for your walk, then reschedule your exercise session for later in the day. If your health club is so crowded in the mornings that you have to wait a half hour to use the stationary bike, look for another gym or try exercising at another time of day.

Enlist the support of your friends and family. Discuss with your family the importance to you of sticking with your exercise program, and that it may require some juggling of schedules. Ask them to be understanding when you get up early to exercise.

- ### *TALK TO YOURSELF*
- On days when you really don't feel like exercising, try talking
- yourself into at least putting on your workout clothes and
- getting out the door. Then encourage yourself to make it
- down the driveway or to the end of the block. You'll find that,
- on most days, once you've started moving you'll feel like
- going on. If you still can't get yourself to complete your
- workout, go back home and, instead of criticizing yourself,
- congratulate yourself for the attempt and try again tomor-
- row.

One woman I had recommended an exercise program for had a tough time with her family about it. She had decided to take a dance aerobics class after work on Mondays, Wednesdays, and Fridays, but this meant that her daughter would have to find another ride to cheerleading practice and her family would get dinner forty-five minutes late on those days. No one supported her efforts to exercise—instead, they made fun of her for trying: "My husband told me I was crazy to parade around in front of my class in my leotard and shorts and the kids told their friends they were starving because 'Mom's too old and fat to be out jumping around and calling it dancing.' I felt so bad that I stopped going to the class."

I told her that she shouldn't let her family prevent her from taking care of herself. We discussed how she could talk to her husband and kids and try to help them understand that she needed their support. However, as hard as she tried to convince them, nothing seemed to get them to change their attitude. So we took another tack and discussed how she could find support from her aerobics instructor—who thought she was doing quite well for a beginner—and the other members of her class in lieu of encouragement at home.

I remember another family situation, however, in which the children and spouse were initially critical of their mother's attempts to incorporate exercise into her schedule. Months of mockery led to a major family discussion about the issue, during which it was decided that the whole family should undertake an exercise program that would be stimulating to all of them. Believe it or not, they took up ice skating. The mother, father, and children, starting out knowing nothing about ice skating, became expert skaters. They learned to love the sport and got a good aerobic workout on a regular basis. Not only did the gastrointestinal problems of the mother improve, but the overall family relationship was strengthened by their regularly doing something they loved together. Other family exercises could include in-line skating or swimming.

Don't Let Boredom Strike

To avoid becoming bored with your workouts, develop a repertoire of several types of exercise that you enjoy so you can vary your activities. Some people do well by walking on Mondays, Wednesdays, and Fridays, swimming on Tuesdays, Thursdays, and Saturdays, and going for a bike ride on Sundays. Others need variety every day, so they jog and then cool off with a swim in the pool.

FRIENDS TO THE RESCUE

Encourage family members to exercise with you—but don't be dismayed if they refuse or even try to sabotage your success. If that happens, look for another workout partner with whom you can exercise together or join an aerobics class or gym where you can find a network of support.

Some of my patients have found that they exercise better when they use music to keep themselves entertained. If you want to add music to your workouts, pick a peppy tune with a beat that will keep you moving briskly. If you're using a treadmill or stair-climbing machine, wear headphones and tune your Walkman to some fast music—not to the news, a talk show, or stock quotations, which will slow you down rather than speed you up.

When you're walking outdoors, try humming a lively tune to yourself—perhaps one you learned years ago at summer camp—or chant inside your head, "Left, left. Left, right, *left,*" as soldiers do.

WRITTEN RECORD

Record your workouts in your journal. Be sure to record the time you exercised, the type of activity you engaged in, and how you felt afterward.

I had one patient, a financial analyst, who was bent on working out at the gym on the most strenuous pieces of equipment, which worked both the arms and legs vigorously, but with his Walkman tuned to the stock reports he was never able to get his heart rate up. I suggested that he switch stations and listen to some fast music with a lively beat. Once he had done that, he began exercising at a pace that made his workouts worthwhile.

Another tool found at health spas and in some patients' backyards can be useful in reducing some unpleasant gastrointestinal symptoms. Many of my patients who use exercise as part of their daily routine reduce the amount of gas, bloating, distention and cramping by spending some time in a Jacuzzi. The beneficial effect of the warm water often lessens the amount of abdominal cramping that some patients, especially those with irritable bowel syndrome, experience. I have one such patient, a middle-aged woman. As she has aged, her irritable bowel syndrome has remained a constant problem, although with exercise, moderate dietary alterations, and the use of charcoal tablets (for more information on charcoal tablets, see chapter 6), she has greatly reduced her symptoms. She joined a gym and, after each daily session on the treadmill, spends ten to fifteen minutes in a warm Jacuzzi. There is little doubt that this has helped lessen her abdominal cramping and bloating.

If you have access to a Jacuzzi, you may want to add this pleasant and possibly beneficial routine to the end of your exercise sessions.

CROSS-TRAIN

Try combining different types of aerobic exercises into your routine. This strategy is called cross-training. For example, you may choose to walk or swim when the weather permits, and work out on a stationary exercise bike indoors when the weather is bad.

Physical Activity in Bits and Pieces

Try to make your workouts a habit, but be flexible. If you miss an exercise opportunity, work physical activity into your day another way. In addition to planning regular aerobic exercise activities into your schedule, there are other ways to "sneak" extra exercise into your day. Instead of looking for the closest parking spot, park your car a few blocks away from the office or at the farthest end of the parking lot at the mall (where your car doors will benefit—they won't get scratched by other cars!). If you're the only one on the escalator, treat it like a staircase and walk up the steps. Walk to the mailbox. Walk your child to the school bus stop instead of driving.

Experiment with "old-fashioned" ways of doing things, such as cutting the lawn with a manual mower or making low-fat frozen yogurt in the kind of ice-cream machine (with a hand-crank) your grandparents used at family picnics. Knead bread. Mop floors. Start a garden. Rake leaves, prune, dig, and pick up trash.

Walk or bike to the corner market instead of always taking the car. Instead of having the daily newspaper delivered to your doorstep, walk to the newsstand and buy a paper each morning. Do housework yourself instead of hiring someone else to do it. Wash your own car instead of using a drive-through car wash. Hide the remote control. Instead of asking someone to bring you a drink, get up and get it yourself.

If you take public transportation to work, get off the bus a few blocks early and walk the rest of the way. At work, brainstorm project ideas with a coworker while taking a walk at lunchtime instead of sitting in the conference room. Stand up when talking on the telephone. Forget your schoolteachers' admonitions to "sit still"—jiggle your leg or tap your foot while you sit at your desk and ponder a dilemma. Take the stairs instead of the elevator—or get off a few floors early and take the stairs the remainder of the way. Use the rest room on another floor and take the stairs to get there. Walk around your building for a break during the workday or during lunch. If your company has a sports team, join it. If not, consider starting one.

If you travel a lot for business, walk while waiting for the plane at the airport. Stay at hotels with fitness centers or swimming pools. Ask the concierge for walking directions to a nice restaurant instead of always hopping into a taxi.

Look for opportunities to increase your physical activity during your leisure time, too. Get out and play catch or tag with your kids—or the neighbors' kids—or race them to the corner—they'll think you're great! Plan family outings and vacations that include exercise, such as hiking, backpacking, and swimming. Consider learning a new sport on your vacation, such as attending a tennis camp or taking surfing lessons. See the sights in new cities by walking, jogging, or biking. At the beach, instead of sitting and watching the waves, get up and walk, play Frisbee, or volleyball, or run around flying a kite. At a picnic, join in on badminton instead of croquet or just eating. At the lake, rent a rowboat or canoe instead of a motorboat. When golfing, walk instead of riding in a cart. Play singles tennis or racquetball instead of doubles. Dance—with someone or by yourself. If you don't know how, take dancing lessons.

Tune the radio to a station that plays upbeat, invigorating music so you'll be encouraged to sing, shake your hips, play an imaginary electric guitar along with the band, or move your arms as if you're conducting the orchestra. Remember that any increase in activity helps—not in place of your regular aerobic workout but as a powerful addition to it.

TAKE TURNS

If taking care of small children or an elderly relative keeps you housebound a good deal of the time, try negotiating with your spouse or a neighbor for an exercise "time swap." Perhaps you could watch a neighbor's children after school for an hour two times a week until the parent gets off work in exchange for an hour of baby-sitting later in the evening or on the weekends while you work out. Or you and your spouse could arrange to take turns working out—one of you in the morning and one in the evening, for example—while the other handles responsibilities at home.

Make an Appointment to Exercise

Schedule your exercise time on your business calendar and treat it as any other important appointment. One of my patients, a sixty-year-old public relations account executive with heartburn, reported that this worked quite well for him. He chose to work out at the gym every day at lunchtime, so he blocked off the time from noon to 1:30 P.M. on his calendar and told his secretary not to schedule any appointments during that time. If a business client wanted to meet with him over lunch, the secretary would simply state that he was booked up at that time, and would suggest that the client come in at another time. This strategy provided another benefit—by avoiding many business lunches, my patient was better able to stick to his diet and avoid alcohol.

Another of my patients has the habit of setting the alarm on his Palm Pilot to go off at a certain time each day, signaling that it's time for his daily workout. When the alarm sounds, he stops whatever he's doing, excuses himself from his colleagues, and heads off to the gym. Most of his coworkers assume he's attending to a business matter, but even those who know where he's going admire his dedication to health and fitness. His work most likely benefits from his exercise breaks, too, as he returns with a clear mind to face the day's challenges.

Scheduling personal time on your business calendar is an important concept for many of my patients. I generally ask that businesspeople block out these times and consider them sacred for exercise, yoga, meditation, or other types of lifestyle improvements.

Once you get into the habit of incorporating more physical activity into your daily life, you'll find that you look at exercise in a whole new light. Over time, you're likely to begin to relish your daily workout instead of considering it a dreaded chore, and you'll start to naturally enjoy getting moving. It's likely that you'll begin to identify with athletes and other exercisers rather than with couch potatoes. And when something comes up that could be a barrier to your daily exercise session, you'll find a way to hurdle the obstacle instead of using it as a convenient excuse to skip your workout. Plus, you're apt to start trying to sell the idea of exercising to others.

One of my patients who had resisted starting an exercise program reported that he now looks forward to jogging in the evenings even more than he used to look forward to coming home and having a few beers. "It's amazing how I can come home so tired and then be revived after my run," he told me. "Whatever is eating at me during the day—an irate phone call from a customer, an unpaid bill, or a meeting that didn't go the way I wanted it to—seems to disappear once I've covered a mile or two."

Exercise is a great way to relieve the stresses of everyday life, and can help you manage GI symptoms that are triggered by stress. But there are other ways to handle non-food triggers, too. We'll talk about these in the next chapter.

5

The Big Picture:
Managing Life Outside Your Digestive System

....

Do you feel your stomach knot up when you hear your in-laws are coming to dinner? Do you feel queasy when you're asked to deliver a report at work? Do social situations like cocktail parties trigger bloating, diarrhea, abdominal pain, or other symptoms? Do you drink pots of coffee and smoke packs of cigarettes when you're working or studying late at night? If you answered "yes" to any of these, then you're being affected by stress.

We don't live in a vacuum. We live in a real world that's full of people, places, and situations that cause stress. As we discussed in chapter 2, everyone likes to maintain the status quo and avoid change. That's because stress occurs whenever there's a significant change in your normal routine. It doesn't matter whether the change is for the worse or for the better. Getting a raise or promotion is stressful—just as getting fired from your job is. Plus, anticipating a change in your normal routine can cause stress. So if you spend a lot of time worrying about "what ifs," you're likely undergoing stress. Speculative changes—that is, things you worry might happen—can cause just as much stress as real changes.

Everyone faces a multitude of stressors every day, but not everyone reacts to them the same way. In people with certain digestive problems, especially irritable bowel syndrome, symptoms such as cramps and abdominal pain can become much worse during periods of stress. If you are one of these people whose gut-wrenching symptoms are triggered by stress, it is most important for you—and those who live and work with you—to realize that you are not "bringing the symptoms on yourself," nor is your condition "all in your mind." You are not a hypochondriac and your condition is not the result of a personality disorder. Your disease is real, and it is affected by stress and how well you cope with it.

In this chapter, I'll give you practical advice for talking to others—including family members and friends, as well as your primary care physician—about your condition. I'll suggest methods of addressing stressful situations and unhealthy relationships with a boss, coworker, or family member who may trigger your digestive symptoms. We'll also discuss a host of other stress-relieving tactics that may help improve your symptoms.

The goal is to help you find relief from your symptoms by increasing your ability to deal with—not avoid—the people and situations that cause them. For example, irritable bowel syndrome patients often experience a flare-up following stressful encounters with difficult bosses, family members, or romantic partners. In trying to avoid this stress, some patients have developed extreme lifestyles in which they avoid difficult situations in life. I strongly recommend that you not do this.

While you may not be able to walk away from a stressful job or family situation, you will likely find that there are many other stress inducers in your life that you *can* change. Later in this chapter, we'll discuss ways that you may sometimes unknowingly contribute to your own stress. By learning to apply certain tactics to your everyday life, such as managing your time better, asserting yourself and saying no, and delegating (or "farming out" to a professional service) job-related or household responsibilities, you may be able to reduce the amount of stress you're feeling.

In addition, I'll show you how to induce the *relaxation response*, a meditative technique that helps you let go of stress. I suggest that GI sufferers do this often to counteract the often unconsciously self-induced stress response and regain a sense of control over their minds and their health.

Many of my patients use yoga to reduce stress in their lives. Yoga is considered a system of exercises to promote control of the mind and body. A well-rounded yoga routine involves the interconnectedness of body, breathing, and mind in a sequence of exercises (positions, or poses, called *asanas*), breathing techniques, and meditation. For more information, see Resources at the end of the book.

Stress Is All Around Us

Stress is produced by everyday events as well as by major life crises. While the death of a spouse, divorce, and loss of a job are understandably stressful, so are holidays, traffic tickets, and going on a date. Even welcomed, happy events, like a new and better job, are stressful. The little hassles of daily life—the car that won't start, the long line at the post office, the boss who leans over your shoulder, the neighbor who plays the stereo loudly while he works in his garage—can also be sources of stress. The accumulated effect of these seemingly minor stressors can have a big impact on your digestive tract. Learning to work with stress is a task for everyone, but it's especially important for people with GI problems. The emotional and physiological roller-coaster of stress wears out the most vulnerable systems first. Thus, an individual whose Achilles' heel is the digestive tract may develop heartburn, cramps, diarrhea, or stomach pain at the first sign of stress.

It's easier to understand why this happens when we realize that there are nerves that travel throughout the digestive system, and that in periods of emotional distress the nervous system is overloaded. The colon is controlled in part by the nervous system, and too much stress can worsen the muscle spasms in the walls of the bowel in people with irritable bowel syndrome. Stress can also cause the production of extra acid in the stomach, suggesting that ulcer pain might be increased by stress, too. By increasing the production of gastric acid, stress can also enhance the amount of acid reflux in heartburn or gastroesophageal reflux disease (GERD). Many studies have shown that the symptoms of inflammatory bowel disease, ulcerative colitis, and Crohn's disease seem to be worse during periods of stress. Indeed, it is my belief that stress can worsen or aggravate almost any gastrointestinal symptom or condition.

The Stress Response

Whether confronted with a frightful event—such as seeing a car suddenly pull out in front of you, or an ongoing tension in your life, such as dealing with a difficult boss—your body's physical response to the stressor is similar.

A hormone called corticotropin-releasing factor (CRF) stimulates the pituitary gland in your brain to release adrenocorticotropic hormone (ACTH). This signals your adrenal glands, near your kidneys, to release more hormones, including adrenaline (also known as epinephrine) and cortisol. Epinephrine and cortisol prepare your body to respond to stress. Your heart beats faster, breathing quickens, and blood pressure rises. Blood is redirected to organs such as your brain and muscles that need oxygen and nutrients to deal with stress. Less blood goes to your stomach—which may be responsible for GI symptoms—and skin. Your body gears up to "fight"—face the challenge—or "take flight," that is, muster up the strength to move out of harm's way. In fact, your body reacts the same way whether the stress is physical or emotional, real or imagined. Think for a minute about how your body reacts when you watch a scary movie. The hair on the back of your neck will stand up in the movie theater just as it would if you were being physically threatened in real life.

What Matters Is How You *React* to Stress

Everyone is surrounded by pressures, changes, demands, and challenges as part of day-to-day life. But not everyone reacts to them the same way. Two people can be subjected to the same situation—such as being stuck in a traffic jam or having to learn a new software program for work—but it can be much more stressful for one person than the other. So it's not so much the situation, but how you *perceive* it and *react to* it, that determines how much stress you feel. While you may not be able to change the situation that is causing the stress, you can change your perception of that stress and choose a more appropriate response to it.

I can think of one example in which the same stress affected two members of the same family quite differently. In that family, both the husband, Tom, and his wife, Linda, have irritable bowel syndrome. Without any real warning, Tom and Linda learned that their twenty-six-year-old son was addicted to cocaine. Neither parent had any suspicion that their son had been using drugs for almost a decade. However, when he was hospitalized because of a drug over-dose, it was clear that drug addiction had been a major part of his life for quite a long time.

Both parents were stressed by the problems related to their son's addiction, but the stress clearly affected one of them more than it did the other. When Tom felt stressed, he played racquetball with his best friend. He'd work through his sadness and anger by throwing himself into the game, running fast and hitting the ball hard. Afterward, he'd sometimes discuss his problems with his buddy, whose now-grown children had given him cause to worry, too, over the years. The combination of exercise and support from a trusted friend helped Tom cope with his problem. His irritable bowel syndrome remained stable and his symptoms neither worsened nor improved.

In contrast, Linda became severely depressed and anxious and the symptoms of her irritable bowel syndrome became especially bad. She had severe abdominal cramps, excessive gas, and severe diarrhea alternating with severe constipation. She worried constantly about her son: *What if he overdoses and doesn't get medical help in time? Why has this happened to her family? Should she have done something different when she was raising him to avoid this?* On one hand, she blamed herself, and on the other she felt victimized and miserable. She wouldn't allow herself to relax or enjoy life.

Eventually, Tom and Linda's son was rehabilitated and now, more than five years later, he is drug-free, productive, and employed. Both parents still have irritable bowel syndrome, but the wife's symptoms improved only after it was clear that her son was recovering. Same stress, but two different reactions from husband and wife, one helpful and the other harmful.

Time-Tested Stress-Relieving Techniques

Over the years I have treated people with various gastrointestinal complaints, I have come to understand that certain tactics can be used to combat stress and to help alleviate symptoms. Here are the stress-relieving techniques I recommend to my patients:

1. Use Your Journal to Track Your Personal Stress Triggers

To help you gain control of your symptoms, you must first play detective. What exactly are the triggers that worsen your symptoms? And—even more important—what can you do about them? That's where your journal comes in. In addition to tracking food triggers, I recommend that you use your journal to keep an inventory of psychological/social triggers that cause you to overeat or repeatedly induce GI symptoms.

Record the time of day when a stressful event occurs, the cause of the stress—such as being stuck in traffic when you were already running late for work, presenting the results of your research to an audience, or arguing with your spouse—as well as any digestive symptom that could be related to the stress, such as tightness in your stomach, indigestion, cramps, constipation, or diarrhea. Over time, your journal will help you become more aware of the stressful events in your day-to-day life that are likely to produce predictable symptoms.

Prior to recording feelings in their journals, some of my patients have been unaware of how much stress they undergo in their daily lives. One patient comes to mind in particular. The first time he came to my office, he arrived a few minutes early and began using the telephone I provide in the waiting room for my patients. When I went to the waiting room to greet him, he was pacing back and forth, holding our office telephone to one ear and his cell phone to the other, apparently carrying on two separate conversations. After he put down one of the phones, he repeatedly checked his watch and glanced over at my secretary. Seeing the situation, I invited him into my office. Right away, I noted that he had a difficult time sitting back and relaxing. Instead, he sat on the edge of his chair, leaned forward, kept shifting his position, and found it difficult to make eye contact as we discussed the worsening of his condition.

He told me he had seen several doctors before coming to me, and that each of them had arrived at the same diagnosis: irritable bowel syndrome. Most of the doctors he had seen had recommended management procedures similar to those I use, with occasional variations. The patient, however, was clearly not pleased with any of the doctors who had preceded me. He seemed to carry the scalps of those doctors on his belt as he scornfully described his interactions with each of them. While doing so, however, he found it difficult to sit still. He crossed then uncrossed his legs; folded then unfolded his arms.

He explained that he did not have time in his busy lifestyle to include any form of exercise. He spoke rapidly and complained of burping and belching, but did not realize that with his rapid speaking he was also swallowing air and contributing to his problems. When I asked him if he felt stressed, he insisted that he experienced no stress during his day-to-day routine. He thought of himself as a highly intelligent, calm, and efficient businessman. It was clear that he had no insight into how much stress he was experiencing—or how that stress was affecting his gastrointestinal symptoms.

Rather than allow my scalp to be added to his collection, I told him I needed some time to think over all the things he had told me and to work out an individualized plan for him that might be of help. I told him I would like to visit with him again the next day or at his earliest convenience. Because of his schedule, his next appointment couldn't take place for a week.

When he returned, once again I observed a scenario similar to the one that had occurred seven days earlier. This time, however, I attempted to point out to him that he had a hard time sitting still and that he tended to sit on the edge of his chair, indicating a high level of stress. I also told him that he spoke rapidly, and that, in doing so, he swallowed air that contributed to his symptoms of belching and abdominal bloating, and that the gas itself might trigger additional discomfort. As we talked, he began to recognize himself in the picture I was painting.

I asked him to use a journal to write down the stressful situations that triggered his uncomfortable symptoms. He did and later admitted he just hadn't realized how much stress had been affecting his life—and his symptoms—until he started keeping track of what was going on before and during their occurrence. For example, he discovered that having lunch at his desk nearly always triggered symptoms. By not getting away from his office for lunch, he continued answering e-mails and phone calls, and never had a chance to stop thinking about work. Consequently, his stomach churned and he frequently began feeling bloated before he had finished his meal, so he ended up throwing out the second half of his sandwich. We talked about the advantages of taking a break from his work while eating, and he agreed to start walking to the cafeteria—*without* his cellular phone—for lunch.

He also agreed to try to follow a new regimen that I generally advise most of my patients to follow. I told him that I felt strongly that exercise would not only help him handle his gastrointestinal symptoms, but would allow him to handle his stress in a more effective manner. I asked him to gradually adopt a program of daily aerobic exercise, starting initially with only a few minutes a day but progressively increasing with the goal of an hour of aerobic exercise each day. He agreed to take a four-day weekend away from his telephone and e-mail every eight weeks and a two-week vacation away from business affairs every six months. I suggested that, rather than expressing anger and frustration inappropriately when a difficult situation occurs, he go for a walk or get involved in some other form of physical activity for stress reduction. He found it difficult to adapt to these changes, but I presented it to him as a challenge. He accepted the challenge—and eventually it worked.

WARNING SIGNS

While some people are well aware when they are experiencing high levels of stress, others have trouble recognizing when they're undergoing chronic everyday stress. If you're unsure about whether you're stressed, ask yourself if you're experiencing any of the following stress warning signs:

- Smoking more?
- Eating more junk foods?
- Drinking more alcohol?
- Feeling angry?
- Having trouble concentrating, making decisions, or getting things done?

2. Begin—and Stick With—a Regular Physical Exercise Program

As discussed in chapter 4, exercise is one of the best ways to manage stress and relieve depression, both of which compromise gastrointestinal health in those with sensitive digestive systems. Because it helps relieve stress, exercise may decrease the pain associated with ulcers and the symptoms of irritable bowel syndrome. The decrease in adrenaline production that occurs naturally after exercise may counteract the stress response.

Those people who have trouble unwinding after work without the help of alcohol may find that exercising at the end of the day helps them relax and lessens their dependence on alcohol as a tranquilizer.

Remember the patient I told you about in chapter 4 who had initially resisted starting an exercise program? He now looks forward to jogging in the evenings even more than he used to look forward to coming home and having a few beers: "Whatever is eating at me during the day—an irate phone call from a customer, an unpaid bill, or a meeting that didn't go the way I wanted it to—seems to disappear once I've covered a mile or two."

Exercise is a great way to relieve the stresses of everyday life, and can help you manage GI symptoms that are triggered by stress.

GET PHYSICAL

If you're feeling stressed, take an exercise break. Go for a walk, head for the gym, or pull weeds in the garden. Physical activity can help you work through the stress before it attacks your digestive tract.

169

3. Learn to Manage Your Time Better

Do you always underestimate how long it will take to get to a destination? Do you always think a task will take less time than it does? If so, you may constantly be stressed over being late or not meeting deadlines and may benefit from learning a variety of time management techniques. Plus, those people who insist that they can't fit regular physical workouts into their daily schedule may be surprised to find plenty of time if they do an honest, careful assessment of how they are actually spending the hours in their days.

I remember a young patient named Carol who worked long hours in a real estate office and then hurried home to take care of two grade-school children. She was always running late, and always seemed to have too many things to do. "I'm always in a rush," she complained to me. "I don't know how other working moms handle everything—preparing meals, checking the kids' homework, making brownies for the school bake sale, and picking up the dry cleaning. And some of my friends do all that and fit aerobics classes into their schedule, too. What's wrong with me that makes me unable to do it all?" I assured Carol that no one really "does it all"—it just may seem that way. I suggested what might help her most is to polish her time management skills: Learn to prioritize tasks, set reasonable goals, and delegate some tasks to others.

Here are some basic time-management techniques that my patients have found helpful:

Keep a time-management log. For one week, try to write down everything you do with your time from the minute you get up until you go to bed. It's a useful exercise just to help you understand how much time routine tasks actually take, but it can also point out how much of your evening is spent surfing the Internet or watching sitcoms on TV.

Prioritize your tasks. Most people find that their tasks fall into three categories: (1) tasks that *must* be done, (2) tasks that must be done, but could be done by someone else, and (3) tasks that don't necessarily have to be done at all.

Among those tasks that you feel you must do yourself, tackle the difficult ones during the time of day when you are most productive—such as first thing in the morning. Schedule your easy tasks for times of the day when you tend to feel low on energy or motivation. For those tasks that could be done by someone else, see my discussion about delegating in technique no. 4 below.

You may be surprised to see how many tasks fall into the category of ones that don't have to be done at all. For example, what's the worst that would happen if the car didn't get washed or the laundry didn't get folded this weekend? You may be causing yourself unnecessary stress by simply having a "to do" list that's too long. Congratulate yourself for every task that you can eliminate altogether from your list.

Set realistic goals and deadlines, and plan projects accordingly. Now that your time log has helped you have a better idea of how much time various tasks actually take, be sure that you schedule enough time for them. Don't allow yourself to be talked into a deadline that you know is unreasonable.

4. Delegate—or "Farm Out" to a Professional Service—Some of Your Job-Related or Household Responsibilities

Do you do mundane chores yourself—either at home or at work—that you could easily delegate to someone else? At times, it may be worth it for you to pay a professional service to pick up and deliver your dry cleaning so you don't have to make an extra stop, transcribe the taped proceedings of a meeting so you don't have to type them up, or cater a party so you don't have to cook. Check the Yellow Pages in your area to see how many services are available, from dog-walking to mobile car detailing to news clipping services. In some cases, you may discover that the professional can do the job quicker and more cheaply than you could do it yourself.

At home, consider asking other members of the family to take on some of the responsibilities you mistakenly thought only you could do, such as shopping for groceries, packing school lunches, balancing the checkbook and paying the bills, or taking care of the family pet. At work, too, you may be able to help your subordinates grow by giving them certain responsibilities you previously thought you had to handle yourself.

Carol, the patient I mentioned earlier who bemoaned the fact that she just couldn't "do it all," learned that brownies from the local bakery sold just as well as homemade ones in the school bake sale. And she found that her husband didn't mind picking up his own dry cleaning on the way home from the office. She enlisted the help of the kids in setting the table and making the salad for dinner, and even got them to help pack their own school lunches. Carol discovered that she had enough time now to take that aerobics class she had been wanting to attend.

5. Learn to Assert Yourself and Say No in a Friendly but Firm Manner

When asked to take on additional responsibilities or chores, some people just can't decline, even when they don't have the extra time or energy. If you're the one the whole family turns to whenever they need free baby-sitting, a cake baked for a fund-raiser, or a book returned to the library, you may be feeling stressed by having to do everyone else's chores on top of your own.

One of my patients, a fifty-four-year-old working grandmother named Pat, was constantly busy doing extra chores for her church and charitable organizations. It seemed like everyone in town—and maybe some in neighboring towns, too—had Pat's phone number and knew that she could always be counted on to take on another project, whether it was sewing costumes for the children's play, editing a newsletter, or phoning for donations. "Whenever they say, 'We always know we can count on you, Pat,' I just feel so guilty if I say no," she told me. I helped her understand that sometimes saying no—politely but firmly—is healthy, and her own health depends on not taking on commitments she can't handle. Once she started saying no, she found it easier to do. "I thought they'd hate me," she said, "but they don't. I think they even respect me more for not being such a pushover."

By learning to set limits for yourself and to politely

communicate those limits to your family and friends, you can avoid unnecessary stress. You may be surprised to see how sympathetically people will respond when you explain that you're just too busy to take on another chore. After all, they're busy, too—that's why they're asking you for help.

If you're out of practice in saying no, here are a few ways to phrase it when you decline to do a requested task:

- "I'd love to help you out, but I'm all booked up."
- "I'm sorry. I can't do it this time."
- "I have another commitment. I hope you find someone who can help you."

At work, when your boss asks you to undertake a project that you don't feel you have time for, politely remind him or her of your existing responsibilities and ask for help in prioritizing which of the projects you should handle first. You'll likely find that your boss simply didn't realize how much else you had to do. If, however, your boss still expects you to take on additional tasks consistently without extra help, you may want to consider looking for less stressful job options.

6. Learn How to Live within Your Financial Means

Finances or money problems are often named as major sources of stress among my patients, particularly for the breadwinners of the family. Too many people get themselves into credit card debt and fail to save for retirement. If you find yourself using one credit card to pay for the bill of another card, you're setting yourself up for major financial stress.

Begin gaining control of your budget by taking inventory of where your money is going. Keep track of every dollar you spend—from the $4.25 you spend for the latte, bagel, and newspaper you pick up on your way into the office each morning to the $49.75 you spend taking the family to a movie—with sodas, candy, and popcorn—on Friday nights. It's likely that you'll find plenty of painless ways to trim your budget, such as by having a healthy breakfast at home or renting videos instead of taking the whole family to a movie theater.

Cut up excess credit cards and avoid paying for luxury items on credit. Instead, save up for them and enjoy anticipating their arrival. Plus, in some cases, by the time you've saved enough money to buy the desired item, you may have changed your mind about wanting it.

If your finances are in especially bad shape, a credit counseling service or financial planner may be able to help you find your way out of debt and start saving for the future by practicing better money management techniques.

A good example of how credit cards can cause stress is the story of a thirty-six-year-old man with gastroesophageal reflux disease (GERD) whom I have been treating. In the natural course of his illness, his symptoms came and went—there were times when they were severe, but there were also long periods when he felt okay. It was clear, however, that external stress, as well as the extremes of emotion, such as anger or depression triggered his symptoms and seemed to increase the frequency of his attacks.

The connection between stress and his symptoms was especially obvious when he developed problems in his business and started to use his credit cards to cover his personal needs as well as his business cash flow problems. Eventually, he was using credit cards to pay off the minimum monthly payments required on other credit cards. As his stress level increased, he tended to smoke more and more cigarettes. Tobacco has been shown to increase the severity of symptoms in GERD. He was on a spiraling downhill course. The more he used credit to pay off credit card debt, the more he smoked and the worse his symptoms got. As he became more and more ill, he became less and less able to cope with his physical problems as well as with his emotional and business problems. Amazingly, he did not realize the role of stress in his overall situation. It was only after I raised the issue of sources of stress in his life that he revealed his business failures, his use of credit cards, his inability to cover the entire debt, and his increasing rate of smoking in order to reduce his anxiety. I was able to show him how one thing led to another, eventually worsening his underlying physical illness. With credit counseling, he was able to develop a payment plan to overcome his immediate financial problems. He reduced the size of his business overhead by moving his business to a less expensive location and by reducing his workforce. He began a smoking cessation program as well as a progressive aerobic exercise program. All of this took about six months, but it was well worth it. The quality of his life improved, and he was able to build an even stronger business and adopt a more fulfilling lifestyle.

For some people, the stress involved in trying to maintain a certain economic lifestyle causes digestive symptoms. I remember another of my patients, a well-to-do stockbroker named Randy whose heartburn flared whenever he was stressed. Randy reduced the stress he was experiencing in life by reassessing his priorities, reframing his idea of success, and making a major lifestyle change. While he enjoyed plenty of money and prestige as a stockbroker, he realized that his hectic job was taking him away from what he really loved—working with young people. He found a job as a teacher at a small parochial school and began living a simpler, slower-paced, more meaningful life. In his new, more pleasurable career, Randy rarely experiences the heartburn pain that so often used to send him running to the medicine cabinet.

7. Take Time Out for Hobbies or Activities You Find Calming

Do you feel that you have no time for activities you used to enjoy, such as reading mystery novels or playing a musical instrument? Do you spend as much time with friends as you used to?

I recommend that my patients observe a Sabbath—that is, take one day off each week for rest and recreation—and that they take vacations. In fact, I recommend a four-day weekend every eight weeks and a two-week vacation every six months for those people who can arrange it. For those people who can't do this—because of logistics such as child care, money, or the kind of work they do—I recommend that they at least try to arrange some sort of relaxing diversion from the routine, such as sending the children to Grandma's so that the husband and wife can enjoy some time together without having to deal with the kids. Not every vacation means getting on a plane and spending a lot of money, either. Some of the most relaxing vacations are spent right at home with a couple of good books and a nice lounge chair in the backyard.

Remember the businessman who couldn't sit still when he first came to my office, and who was so tied to his stressful job that he needed to talk on two telephones at once in my office waiting room? Learning to take long weekends and real vacations did him a world of good. The concept of being "out of touch" was difficult for him to accept at first. But he gradually weaned himself from picking up office voice-mail messages or checking his business e-mail on weekends, and from calling the office while on vacation "just to see that everything was all right." The key to relaxation is truly *letting go*.

PERSONAL DAY

If you've been feeling especially stressed lately, take a "personal" day off from work to recharge. Do something you wouldn't ordinarily do, such as going to a movie matinee or driving to the country. By paying attention to times when your body needs a "time-out," you'll be able to return to work refreshed and more productive, and may avoid painful episodes when your digestive symptoms flare up.

8. Reduce Your Worry-Related Stress and Negative Thoughts

Do you worry a lot about endless stressful possibilities, such as:

- What if I oversleep and miss the test?
- What if I lose my job?
- What if I get really sick and can't work to pay the bills?

If so, odds are that you're worrying about a lot of things that will never actually happen. And even if they were to happen, worrying about them won't help solve anything. You can reduce your stress by taking positive steps to avoid the dreaded event, such as setting an extra alarm clock to avoid oversleeping, keeping in touch with business colleagues at other companies for potential job referrals if you should need them, and looking into long-term disability insurance should you become too sick to work. Translate free-floating anxieties into a concrete plan of action.

WORKING WITH WORST-CASE SCENARIOS

Another healthy way to overcome stress related to worrisome situations is by planning how you would handle it if the situation did occur, and then quit worrying about it. You'll know that you have a plan of attack just in case the worst possibility does happen. Ask yourself, "If I'm late, what's the worst thing that will happen?" and "If that does happen, what steps could I take to rectify the situation?"

Automatically thinking negative or catastrophic thoughts is another pitfall that causes many people unnecessary stress. Examples of negative thinking include:

- "I'll never get the job."
- "There's no way a woman like her would ever go out with a loser like me."
- "I won't ever be able to lose thirty pounds."

REALITY CHECK

Catastrophic thinking occurs when you blow a small incident out of proportion, such as thinking you'll be fired just because you made a minor mistake. If you find yourself thinking negative or catastrophic thoughts, try to force yourself to stop and reassess how well your thoughts fit with reality. Are you exaggerating the negative and contributing to your own stress? Smile as you ask yourself, "C'mon, now—is it really all that bad?" Watch out for thoughts that include words like "always" and "never."

Another patient I treated with irritable bowel syndrome was a physician. When he was my patient, he was in his forties and had had his irritable bowel syndrome for over twenty years. When he had been in med school, like so many other young medical students, he frequently thought he had the symptoms of whatever disease he was currently studying. During periods of stress, such as prior to examinations, his irritable bowel syndrome would become especially severe. Diarrhea alternating with constipation, abdominal cramps, gas, and bloating would increase progressively as the test drew nearer, and then would magically improve the day after the exam.

Later in life, his tendency to speculate about his own health and to worry about worst-case scenarios increased. When he experienced pain in his lower back after lifting weights, he immediately worried, *"What if I have a ruptured disk? Or what if it's cancer of the pancreas?"* His symptoms of irritable bowel syndrome became worse, and he worried, *"What if I have colon cancer?"* None of his "what ifs" came true, but his fears of new diseases and conditions caused him unnecessary stress and anxiety—which in turn made his symptoms of irritable bowel syndrome more severe and more frequent. Had he promptly arranged to have the appropriate tests done to rule out each potential disease, he might have avoided years of needless stress and suffering.

9. Hone Your Communication Skills

Human relationships by nature are infinitely complicated and can be further challenged by a disorder that requires a certain degree of compassion and sensitivity. Nothing impacts our emotional lives as profoundly as our close relationships, and many GI disorders, especially irritable bowel syndrome, are so closely linked to our emotional state that the importance of maintaining healthy relationships and open channels of communication cannot be overemphasized. Here are some basic strategies for good communication:

Listen closely to the person with whom you're speaking. Don't plan what you'll say next while she's talking. Instead, try to "put yourself in the other person's shoes" and understand her point of view. When she's finished talking, try repeating back, "So you're saying that you feel..." to be sure that you got it right. By showing that you are genuinely trying to understand her perspective, you also encourage the other person to listen carefully when it's your turn to speak.

Express your feelings constructively. Say, "I feel (angry, hurt, upset, etc.) when you (fail to acknowledge my contributions, don't phone to say that you'll be home late, forget my birthday, etc.).” Statements beginning with “I feel...” are far more effective than those that begin by confronting the other person with an accusatory statement, such as “You never...”

If you are in conflict, don't blame the other person. Try to make him or her feel less defensive or angry by using a nonthreatening approach. For example, if your husband is always late for dinner, calmly explain to him that not knowing when to expect him makes it difficult for you to plan the meal, and that eating too close to bedtime contributes to your nighttime heartburn. Help him understand how you are feeling.

Focus on positive, concrete ways to solve the problem. Enlist the other person's help in outlining a workable win-win strategy. Avoid being sidetracked by revisiting past negative incidents that don't relate to the present problem. For example, once you've explained *why* you are uncomfortable when your husband is late for dinner, together you can decide that it would help if he phones you when he's running late. That way, you can either put the meal on hold for a half hour, or, if the wait is going to be longer, you can go ahead and eat without him.

LEAN ON THEM
Ask friends for support when you need to cope with a stressful situation. An ear to bend and a shoulder to lean on can go a long way toward helping you get through tough times. Plus, in describing your problem to a friend, you may find that you organize your thoughts and gain perspective you didn't have when thinking about the situation all by yourself.

Many of my patients have learned how to interact successfully with strangers and business associates, but those they love or care about are still real sources of stress. One way to improve relations with family and friends is to practice positive communication skills and not expect them to read your mind. Instead of thinking, "She's my mother, she should *know* how I feel," tell her exactly how you *do* feel. Being specific always helps. If you ask your husband for help around the house, don't assume he'll know what you want him to do. His idea of helping around the house might mean simply taking out the garbage each evening, while yours includes giving the baby a bath and putting the dishes in the dishwasher as well. By defining your terms clearly, you'll avoid unnecessary misunderstandings that lead to stressful encounters.

Better communication skills can help resolve job-related conflicts, too. One of my patients discovered through keeping her journal that her symptoms worsened every time she had a meeting with her boss. She left the meetings with lots of questions in her mind: *"Exactly what does she want me to do?" "Didn't she like the job I did on the last project?" "Doesn't she know how I feel about working on the Smith account?"* We discussed ways in which she could improve her communication skills with her boss and she found that these techniques helped both her and her boss to come away from meetings with a clearer understanding of each other's needs and expectations.

Another important rule of effective communication is to avoid jumping to conclusions. Be sure that you don't assume that someone is reacting negatively to you just because he or she hasn't returned your phone call or replied to your e-mail message. Instead of spending hours replaying your message in your mind and thinking how you could have phrased it differently, consider alternate explanations for the person's behavior. Is it possible that he or she is out of town or simply too busy to respond right away?

I have had patients who have made the mistake of jumping to conclusions about their medical condition. Some made assumptions that were inappropriate and denied themselves the benefit of good medical care because of their conviction that a worst-case scenario was taking place. One such patient was a highly successful and respected businessman named Richard. He had accumulated his wealth by a combination of hard work and acting on his own intuition and superior intelligence. While Richard had been able to diagnose the problems of ailing companies and prescribe appropriate fixes for them, his mistake was to assume that he could serve as his own physician. After all, no matter how smart he was, he had never gone to medical school.

When Richard started experiencing abdominal pain after eating, he initially assumed that he had an ulcer. When the pain progressively increased he began losing a great deal of weight—fifty pounds over a ten-month period of time—developed diarrhea, and had foul-smelling, oily stools. He concluded that he had cancer, yet he was so frightened at the prospect that he wouldn't see a doctor to confirm it. He became very depressed and underwent a personality change so severe that he became ineffective in business, nearly stopped communicating at home, and was unable to make any sort of decisions.

During the course of his downward spiral, Richard

finally decided to consult his family physician. Unfortunately, the doctor he chose to see had a very busy practice and found it necessary to drastically limit the time he spent with each patient, so he didn't have time to listen to Richard's somewhat complex and unusual medical history. Instead, the physician, like Richard, assumed that Richard's significant weight loss and increasing abdominal pain were signs of cancer, and he proceeded to run a series of cancer-detecting tests.

Richard had virtually given up hope that there could be any chance he didn't have cancer, but his wife insisted that he consult a specialist for another opinion. That's when he came to see me. As I questioned him carefully, I learned that Richard's pain had started before he began to lose weight, and that the pain occurred only after eating. The larger the meal he tried to eat, the more pain he experienced. Eventually, he stopped eating to avoid the pain he knew he would feel after eating even a small meal.

When I performed a thorough physical examination, I discovered an abnormal sound coming from the blood vessels in Richard's abdomen, and found that his pulse was weak in his legs. It was clear to me that Richard had a vascular disease—hardening of the arteries—that prevented enough blood from getting through to his stomach and intestines. He didn't have cancer after all. I sent him to have an abdominal angiogram—a test that checks to see if blood vessels are open so blood can flow through them properly—to confirm my suspicions, and he then underwent surgery to fix the problem. If Richard had not jumped to the conclusion that he had cancer, and had instead sought appropriate medical help, he could have saved himself many unproductive months of pain, worry, and hopelessness. Plus, he might have been able to avoid surgery by seeing a doctor earlier, being properly diagnosed, and starting a diet and exercise program designed to promote cardiovascular health.

Telling Others About Your Condition

Another communication strategy that may help you reduce some of your stress is learning how to tell others about your GI condition. Do you have trouble explaining the connection between the mind and the gut to your family, friends, or colleagues? To help them understand that the emotions and intestines are interwoven, remind them that nearly everyone has experienced a sensation of having butterflies in the stomach before delivering a speech or has awakened with a bellyache the morning of an important exam. In people who have irritable bowel syndrome, the link between the GI system and emotions may simply be stronger than in most people. Another way of looking at it is that stress affects everyone differently. Some people react to stress by getting a headache or sweaty palms, while other people respond in the gut.

GI sufferers, especially those prone to gas and diarrhea, are often embarrassed about their conditions—even when discussing these matters with their family members. But, unless you tell them the name of your illness and describe its symptoms and how diet, exercise, and stress affect those symptoms, they will have no way of understanding what you are going through and why you are making lifestyle changes. Talk with the children in the family, too, to educate them about your illness and what you are doing to manage your symptoms.

OPEN SECRET

Be sure to tell your loved ones that you don't want or need to be coddled or "handled with kid gloves" because of your condition. Explain that the reason you are telling them about your condition is so that they will understand your need for sticking with your dietary regimen and exercise program, keeping your doctor's appointments, and learning how to manage stress—and that you are counting on them for support and encouragement.

I recently witnessed a classic example of the importance of good communication for a patient with irritable bowel syndrome. Cynthia, a thirty-four-year-old administrative assistant, had experienced irritable bowel syndrome since she had been a teenager. She married Rob in her twenties and raised four children. Throughout her marriage, the symptoms of her irritable bowel syndrome were sometimes worse than others, as the stresses of life came and went. Because Cynthia's symptoms flared up whenever she was upset, Rob began to believe—and tell all their friends—that his wife's condition was "all in her head." He grew distant and unsympathetic. Eventually the couple began to talk of divorce.

Fortunately, they decided to see a therapist first. In couples' therapy, they both learned to frankly express their feelings. He gained a better understanding of the severity of her discomfort and learned that she was not "bringing the symptoms on herself." She got a better understanding of his frustration with having a wife who would predictably develop diarrhea and cramping during a dispute, seemingly as a method of getting out of the argument. It became clear to both of them that stress and anxiety worsened her symptoms, and that his lack of compassion and understanding contributed to that stress and anxiety. They worked together to confront the problem rather than bury it. Over a period of time, he grew more supportive, and her irritable bowel symptoms became less frequent and severe. Improved communication has made their relationship stronger and Cynthia healthier.

10. Practice the Relaxation Response

In 1975, Dr. Herbert Benson of the Harvard Medical School wrote a book called *The Relaxation Response,* in which he described a meditative technique that helps you to downshift all the bodily systems that gear up in stressful situations. The meditation and relaxation training techniques he teaches can help you essentially "let go" of stress.

Benson studied the physiological changes that occur in people during meditation. He found that the changes that take place are the opposite of those that occur when we are stressed. Stress causes your blood pressure to rise, your heart and lungs to work faster, your muscles to tense, and blood to flow to the heart instead of to your hands and feet. Meditation, on the other hand, causes blood pressure to drop, breathing and heart rate to slow, and muscles to relax. Blood flows freely throughout the body, and the extremities become warmer with increased blood flow. Muscles relax and function more normally. Thus, by practicing meditative relaxation techniques, you can help your-self slip into a different physiological state—one that allows you to handle stressful life events in a better way.

Benson pointed out that there are several ways to elicit the relaxation response, and they all involve repetition. The repetition can involve words, sounds, prayer, or even mus-cular activity or movement, such as walking. To elicit the relaxation response, some people pick a word, phrase, or mental image on which to focus. Some of my patients have chosen a word like *peace* or *relax*. Others prefer to picture a pleasant relaxing place, such as a deserted beach or a quiet forest. If using a repeated movement, such as walking, the steady rhythm of the repeated footfalls triggers the relax-ation response.

RELAXATION RESPONSE

To elicit the relaxation response using a repeated word, phrase, or mental picture, sit quietly in a comfortable position with your eyes closed and your muscles relaxed. Breathe slowly, and repeat your word or phrase or picture your image as you exhale. Simply witness the thoughts that pass through your mind, and, if you become distracted, don't worry about it—just return to repeating your word or focusing on your image. Whenever everyday thoughts intrude, let them go, and return to the repetition. Continue for ten to twenty minutes. When you're faced with a stressful situation, this simple exer-cise can have an immediate calming effect.

Benson's work led to a series of findings dealing with mind-body mechanisms that can be used with medically significant impact on various illnesses or disorders.

Although initially considered "alternative medicine" of questionable benefit, Benson's approach is now more widely accepted in much of mainstream medicine, and doctors like me are now recommending it to our patients who suffer from stress-related disorders. We're not sure exactly how it works, but some researchers have suggested that eliciting the relaxation response once or twice a day may block the effects of a hormone called noradrenalin, which plays a key role in the stress response.

LISTEN TO YOUR FOOTSTEPS

Did you know you can trample stress out of your life by putting one foot in front of the other—again, and again, and again? When you walk alone and focus on the repeated sound of your foot hitting the ground, you can trigger the relaxation response. When stray thoughts about work or family problems enter your mind, don't be concerned, instead, simply "let them go," and return your focus to the sound of your footsteps. It probably won't happen on the first try, but be patient and keep trying. Eventually, you will find that you have slipped into a meditative, relaxed state and that you can return to this state any time you step out for a walk.

Often my patients with irritable bowel syndrome tell me that by practicing the relaxation response at the first signs of familiar rumblings in their gut, which they recognize as the beginnings of unpleasant symptoms, they are sometimes able to short-circuit the stress response instead of being forced to retreat to the bathroom with terrible diarrhea and cramping. One such patient, a twenty-eight-year-old sales clerk named Valerie, had begun a walking program for the sole purpose of losing weight. After two months of walking regularly, however, she reported that her walks had become a form of stress therapy. "When I feel my stomach begin to knot up, I drop everything and hit the pavement for a stress-reducing walk. After a couple of laps around the park near my office, I feel so much better," she told me. Valerie was able to stop taking medicines for her irritable bowel syndrome and she lost twenty-five pounds—mostly attributable to her new habit of walking and to calorie reduction.

TAKE A MENTAL VACATION

At stressful times during the day, some of my patients find it helpful to close their eyes for a few minutes and imagine a place of peace and solitude—perhaps a serene beach with waves gently lapping at the shore, a garden path surrounded by blooming flowers, or a quietly bubbling brook in the woods. With practice, they were able to quickly and quietly escape to their own private mental refuge and elicit a calmness and feeling of safety—without ever leaving their home or office or business meeting. The idea isn't to evade the situation that's causing the stress; instead, the inner journey helps stop negative thoughts and replaces them with positive thoughts and feelings. After a few minutes spent in the calm, soothing inner environment, they can return to the real world with a stronger, more positive attitude.

11. Take Time to Play and Laugh—Laughter Is Good Medicine

Scientific studies have shown that just as the relaxation response evokes calming physical effects that are the opposite of those experienced during "fight or flight," laughter can lower blood pressure, slow the heart and breathing rate, and relax muscles. In this way, laughter can help alleviate the physical effects of stress. But laughter can actually do much more.

Bill, one of my patients with irritable bowel syndrome, really took my suggestions about humor to heart. He kept a scrapbook filled with jokes and cartoons he'd clipped from newspapers and magazines in his bottom desk drawer. Whenever he was feeling particularly stressed at work and felt his stomach begin to knot up, he'd close his office door, open his "humor book," and have a good laugh. At home, he kept a supply of old black-and-white slapstick videos to help him relax after a stressful day at work. He even kept some humorous audiotapes of old radio programs in his car for the trip back and forth from the office. Bill also began incorporating a bit of humor into his presentations and memos at work, and found that he could often defuse tension in difficult situations by adding the perspective that humor affords. Plus, he found that people seemed to pay closer attention and remember what he said better when he'd added a touch of humor to his talks. Overall, looking at things from the lighter side helped him communicate better, reduce stress, and eliminate most of his digestive complaints.

Those who suffer from common GI disorders need to deal with their condition in the context of a multitude of outside factors, including improving communication with others, handling unhealthy relationships, understanding the enormous effect of stress on gastrointestinal health, and learning the benefits of relaxation.

We've discussed ways to deal with stress, anxiety, depression, and other triggers that cause you to stray from your healthy eating program. Plus, by following the recommendations set forth in this chapter, I believe that you can minimize the discomfort and inconvenience of your symptoms and begin feeling good most of the time—without resorting to medication.

6

When You Need Medicines
for GI Complaints

....

THROUGHOUT this book, I have discussed ways that people with heartburn, gas, bloating, diarrhea, and constipation can relieve these symptoms through lifestyle changes—without using medicines. However, there are times when medicines *are* needed, either because the patient's condition is quite severe, or because symptoms do not respond to lifestyle modifications alone. There are also cases when patients are not willing or able to make the necessary lifestyle changes, and I am forced to resort to treating them with medications, too. Lastly, there are cases in which GI symptoms indicate a more serious medical condition, such as diverticulitis or Crohn's disease.

Even when I do prescribe medications to my patients, I still place a strong emphasis on lifestyle modifications. In many cases, the medications are only needed for a short time, and then the patient can successfully manage his condition with diet, exercise, and stress-reduction techniques alone. Remember, too, that all drugs have side effects, so we don't want to take them unnecessarily.

Taking drugs for digestive disorders is not always a bad idea, nor is it always a good idea. Each individual patient's case is different, and it takes medical training and common sense to determine whether to manage symptoms with or without drugs. In fact, it also takes careful thought to decide which symptoms should not be addressed at all. That's because we all get aches and pains, gas, bloating, occasional heartburn or indigestion, and burping from time to time. These transient symptoms usually don't require concern or treatment. I worry because, in our society, it is common to overmedicate, and then we often have to deal with the side effects of drugs. In situations in which short-lived symptoms may have spontaneously disappeared without drugs, it seems a waste of time and money and additional physical stress on the body that was likely unnecessary.

WAIT-AND-SEE ATTITUDE

Don't be too quick to reach for the medicine cabinet or drive to the drugstore every time you experience little aches and pains or irregular stools or gassy feelings. Try waiting to see if the symptom will go away by itself. In many cases, it will.

I encountered an example of this situation last year when I cared for a young woman who developed diarrhea during the time that many of her friends and children had developed the same symptom, suggesting that it was caused by a virus. The diarrhea came on at an especially difficult time for her. She had an important new business presentation to make for work the next week and she wanted to be sure that she recovered quickly both to prepare for the big day and do well at the presentation itself.

She stressed to her family doctor the importance of being able to make her presentation, and virtually demanded that he treat her symptoms as completely as possible so as to eradicate the diarrhea before the all-important day. Her doctor advised her to make some simple dietary changes, such as avoiding milk and milk products until the diarrhea spontaneously went away. He pointed out that in many cases of viral diarrhea (diarrhea caused by infection with a virus), people develop a temporary lactose intolerance, and, if this were the case, she would just have to wait a while to see if a milk-free diet would help. He also advised her to avoid foods that stimulate bowel movements, such as those rich in fiber—especially uncooked fruits and vegetables, such as salads.

Nevertheless, she demanded an antibiotic to ensure that she recovered soon. Eventually, in order to appease her, her family doctor agreed to provide her with a common antibiotic. However, unbeknownst to her doctor, the patient was already taking another antibiotic because she had developed a sore throat and a runny nose and had consulted a head and neck doctor. (She had chosen to see a specialist and not her family doctor for her sore throat and runny nose because she thought they might be related to a sinus condition he had treated her for earlier that year.) She was now receiving two antibiotics from two different doctors. Most likely, neither of these antibiotics was necessary because her condition was caused by infection with a virus, and antibiotics don't kill viruses.

To make things even worse, she decided to double the dose of each of her drugs, thinking (as too many people mistakenly think) that she would get better faster. Within a few days, her diarrhea became more severe and recurred throughout the day and night keeping her from sleeping well. She developed cramps and a low-grade fever.

Her family doctor referred her to me, and I ordered a test called a colonoscopy. We found the characteristic signs of antibiotic-associated colitis, a potentially serious condition if allowed to progress. The first thing we did was to stop the antibiotics. Sometimes when this fails, we need to use a different antibiotic to treat the cause of antibiotic-associated colitis, which usually is a bacteria called *Clostridium difficile*. In this case, simply stopping the antibiotics and waiting resulted in total resolution of her diarrhea within three days. Unfortunately, with the onset of her antibiotic-associated colitis, the patient became so sick that she was unable to make her presentation.

Medicines for Heartburn or Gastroesophageal Reflux Disease (GERD)

Let's take a look at the variety of medicines that are available today to treat heartburn or gastroesophageal reflux disease (GERD). Taking nonprescription medicines according to the instructions is safe to relieve occasional heartburn, but it is no substitute for adopting healthier, permanent lifestyle modifications. Far too many people get into the habit of taking over-the-counter medicines on a regular basis in lieu of making the commitment to change their diet and exercise habits and manage stress more effectively.

Antacids, such as Alka-Seltzer®, Maalox®, Mylanta®, Rolaids®, Amphogel®, Alternagel®, Alka-2®, and Tums® work by neutralizing the acid in your stomach. Despite the many brands, they all contain similar ingredients. Some of them (for example, Mylanta) contain magnesium salts, others (for example, Amphogel and Alternagel) contain aluminum salts, and still others (for example, Tums and Alka-2) contain calcium salts. Each of these salts may produce different side effects. The major side effect of taking magnesium salts is diarrhea, while the most common side effect of taking aluminum or calcium salts is constipation. When taken for a very long time, calcium salts can lead to kidney failure in some people, too. These side effects are a good reason not to take antacids for more than 5 or 6 days 3 or 4 times per year.

The class of drugs known as H2 blockers includes brands such as Zantac®, Tagamet®, Pepcid®, and Axid®. These H2 blockers are available in both nonprescription and prescription strengths. They work by reducing the production of acid in the stomach. Like antacids, though, they are only recommended for occasional, not continual, use. Side effects can include headache, diarrhea, dizziness, rash, and nausea. If you are taking H2 blockers, be sure your doctor or pharmacist knows all the medicines you are taking with it. H2 blockers can interact with other medicines you are taking at the same time. Remember that these medicines provide only short-term symptom relief and are not to be used in place of lifestyle modifications.

The medicines that are most effective in treating gastroesophageal reflux disease are called proton-pump inhibitors and are available only with a prescription—although nonprescription strengths of these medications are expected to eventually be available over-the-counter. They inhibit the so-called gastric pump that is required for the stomach's cells to secrete acid, and work by inhibiting the acid-producing cells in the stomach. These two leading proton-pump inhibitors are Prilosec® and Prevacid®. These drugs not only relieve symptoms of severe chronic reflux but also promote healing of the inflamed esophagus, helping avoid complications of prolonged heartburn such as stricture (extreme narrowing of the esophagus), bleeding, and even cancer of the esophagus. I sometimes prescribe these medications for patients with severe heartburn who show signs of esophagitis, such as hoarseness, loss of voice, or chronic coughing. Side effects are rare, but may include an allergic reaction, headache, stomach pain, or diarrhea. The use of these drugs should not serve as an excuse for eating foods that can be harmful even if the drugs mask the symptoms. Alcohol, fatty foods, and spices can promote irritation even in the absence of heartburn.

In many instances, common sense tells me that a patient's symptoms are so severe, significant, or specific that drug treatment must be used from the start, even if the patient has not yet tried to make lifestyle changes.

For example, while most people who have occasional heartburn are likely to respond to the common-sense lifestyle changes (described in earlier chapters), those who have had severe heartburn on a regular basis for many years are often found to have a condition called *erosive esophagitis*. To diagnose this condition, a doctor looks into the esophagus with an endoscope (a kind of thin, flexible tube with a camera lens and a light on the end) in a procedure called an endoscopy. If the doctor sees characteristic inflammatory changes and ulcerations (sores) on the esophagus, he or she knows that this patient has a more serious condition and should begin treatment. Esophagitis can lead to narrowing of the esophagus and to other complications.

A WORD ABOUT OVER-THE-COUNTER ANTACIDS

Many people get into the habit of taking the kind of antacids that can be purchased without a prescription (or "over-the-counter" at a drugstore) quite frequently. These include products such as Tums, Maalox, Mylanta, and DiGel®. These medicines do not buffer as much acid as the drugs that require a prescription from your doctor.

If you find that you're taking these nonprescription medicines often, it's likely that you should be making the kinds of lifestyle changes outlined in this book. If lifestyle changes don't sufficiently reduce your symptoms, then you should talk to your doctor, who may prescribe more powerful drugs at least until your symptoms come under control.

Some over-the-counter antacids, such as Tums and Mylanta, also contain calcium. While a little calcium is a good thing, taking too much calcium (over 500 mg, as can occur when people pop antacid tablets in their mouths all day long) can cause constipation.

I tell my patients whose gastroesophageal reflux disease has progressed to the point at which they show signs of esophagitis to follow all of the common-sense approaches previously described, but I also place them on a proton-pump inhibitor. These medicines help bring the condition rapidly under control and may prevent progression of the illness.

I saw a patient who had spent a good part of his life failing to follow any of the common-sense rules. In his fifties, he was obese, worked under exceptional stress as an air traffic controller, and in the evenings drank wine and mixed drinks. He smoked cigarettes and cigars, and he had never participated in any kind of an exercise program. He enjoyed spicy foods and had become accustomed to multiple daily episodes of heartburn.

WARNING SIGN

If heartburn causes severe discomfort or you have trouble swallowing, be sure to see a doctor. Left untreated, chronic reflux can scar and narrow your esophagus. It can also lead to a condition called Barrett's esophagus, in which the lining of the stomach extends into the lower esophagus. Barrett's esophagus is associated with an increased risk of cancer.

He came to me not because of the heartburn but because for several months he had noted a progressive increased difficulty with swallowing. After listening to his story and realizing he had gone for many years without any form of treatment or lifestyle adjustments, I was concerned that he might have developed a severe narrowing of the esophagus or even cancer of the esophagus. He underwent an upper endoscopy and, indeed, we did find severe narrowing of the esophagus, but fortunately no evidence of cancer. I placed him on a lifestyle modification program together with a proton-pump inhibitor. It was clear that he had esophagitis that had progressed to such a degree that the esophagus was scarred and narrowed. He had severe acid reflux and although lifestyle changes were important, this was a situation where medication was necessary to take care of his problem.

A sixty-year-old college professor came to me because he'd recently experienced a sensation of food "sticking" in the middle of his chest on swallowing and he'd lost thirty pounds over the previous six months. Although he didn't complain of it, I learned in taking his history that he'd had heartburn almost every day for as long as he could remember. In fact, he thought that having heartburn was a normal part of life. To alleviate his symptoms, he would use over-the-counter medication in excessive quantities. Each day he would habitually consume at least one package of Rolaids along with some other antacid tablets. He was amazed that after more than thirty years of this lifestyle, about six months ago, his heartburn seemingly disappeared. He no longer needed Rolaids or antacids, but he was bothered by that sensation of food sticking. His story was characteristic of someone with gastroesophageal reflux disease who develops esophageal cancer. The patient underwent upper endoscopy and it was clear that he did have carcinoma of the esophagus. He was treated with surgery, but he survived only one year. He was one of those people who really did need treatment with drugs, such as proton-pump inhibitors, in order to properly treat his gastroesophageal reflux disease.

Another type of medication, called a prokinetic agent, is also available by prescription. Propulsid® (cisapride) is the main example of this class of drug. These drugs don't affect acid production. Instead, they work by increasing pressure on the lower esophageal sphincter (LES) so that it doesn't open up and let stomach contents seep back into the esophagus. Prokinetic drugs are useful when the esophagus is not yet injured by acid reflux. These drugs can have side effects, and should not be taken by people who have certain medical disorders, such as heart disease or kidney failure. Again, I believe that, for most people, avoiding foods such as peppermint, caffeine, and alcohol that cause the LES to relax can be an effective means of relieving heartburn without having to resort to taking these drugs.

Medications for Irritable Bowel Syndrome (IBS)

The majority of people with irritable bowel syndrome will need no medications if they follow the diet and lifestyle recommendations I have set forth in this book. The only times I prescribe medicines for people with irritable bowel syndrome are when specific symptoms become out of control.

I have a patient, Greta, with irritable bowel syndrome and whose symptoms have always been mild to moderate and often been worsened during periods of stress and anxiety. She has alternating diarrhea and constipation and abdominal cramps. She has found that she can reduce the frequency and severity of her symptoms with aerobic exercise, stress reduction, a diet free of uncooked fruits and vegetables, and patience.

ACTIVATED CHARCOAL TABLETS

Many patients who suffer from gas and bloating have found relief by taking activated charcoal tablets (Charcocaps®). Activated charcoal is an odorless, tasteless product, made by burning wood pulp. Activation occurs as oxidizing gases work at high temperatures. The charcoal has large surface area, which enables it to absorb gas and to convert large gas bubbles into smaller, less noticeable ones. Charcoal tablets can be taken at a dose of up to two tablets four times daily.

While charcoal is effective at reducing gas symptoms, it can also interfere with certain other medicines that a patient might be taking. Therefore, patients taking digitalis preparations, thyroid medications, or certain other medicines should not take activated charcoal at the same time. If you are taking activated charcoal tablets, talk with your doctor about how this remedy might interfere with other medicines you are taking.

However, Greta has an aunt whom I often care for too, whose irritable bowel syndrome has been present for almost forty years. The aunt's episodes are characterized by severe cramping, abdominal pain, and an inability to have bowel movements without great discomfort or frequent diarrhea. Her symptoms greatly affect the quality of her life and virtually make it impossible for her to leave home during these attacks. In contrast to the way I treated her niece, I decided to prescribe an antispasmodic medication for this patient because of the severity and frequency of her symptoms. With an antispasmodic agent, she gets relatively prompt relief of her pain. Then, with the institution of dietary modifications and aerobic exercise, her other symptoms have come under good control. She uses the antispasmodic medicine as needed for her pain, and has been able to keep working and have a social life. However, I manage the niece's symptoms, which are not as severe or frequent, without the use of drugs.

I also treated a patient named Eileen whose crampy abdominal pain due to irritable bowel syndrome is so severe that she finds it intolerable. For the first few months, we tried to alleviate her pain without medication by modifying her lifestyle. Eileen avoided raw fruits and raw vegetables—especially salads and gas-producing vegetables like cabbage, broccoli, and Brussels sprouts. She also took activated charcoal tablets (Charcocaps), which are available over-the-counter and can help alleviate gas.

Eileen also walked for thirty minutes each evening after work. In spite of these measures, her abdominal cramps were still intolerable. That's why I prescribed an antispasmodic agent called Levsin® for her. I directed Eileen to take one or two of these tablets under her tongue whenever she needed them for her cramps, and they provided much relief. (For other patients who experience intolerable cramps every day despite their attempts to alleviate the pain using lifestyle changes, I sometimes prescribe Levsin to be taken three to four times per day.)

Medicines for Diarrhea or Constipation

I sometimes recommend that diarrhea be temporarily treated with an over-the-counter medicine such as Imodium® that may slow gastrointestinal motility. Antispasmodic drugs are also helpful in temporarily treating diarrhea by reducing spasms of the intestines and stomach.

I caution patients experiencing constipation against getting into the habit of using over-the-counter laxatives. It's easy to get into a vicious cycle and become dependent on laxatives, in which you keep taking them more and more. This cycle often occurs because the colon may empty of all fecal material when laxatives are taken and it may take a few days for sufficient material to form for the next bowel movement. People often become worried that this length of time without a bowel movement indicates further constipation, so they take more laxatives.

Instead of laxatives, I recommend bulk-forming agents, such as psyllium (Metamucil®, Perdiem®, Fiberall®, etc.) or methylcellulose (Citrucel®), all of which are available without a prescription. These agents are not laxatives, and therefore can be used regularly. They work by retaining water and will make a hard stool softer.

For patients who alternate between diarrhea and constipation, bulk-forming agents can help control both problems. In addition to making hard stools softer, they can absorb excess water in the gut during times of diarrhea, thus making the stool firmer.

Louise, a sixty-five-year-old retired school principal, was a patient with irritable bowel syndrome who needed medications for her constipation. Louise's IBS was of the type often referred to as "constipation-predominant," because her main symptom was constipation. Louise had silently suffered from IBS for over forty years when she came to see me last year. During her first visit, we discussed possible lifestyle modifications that work for many other people, but it was soon clear to me that Louise had already tried all the usual common-sense measures for alleviating her constipation. She went for a walk every day for exercise. She had tried eating a high-fiber diet, including foods like prunes and prune juice, and had even tried supplementing her high-fiber diet with psyllium (Metamucil), but her constipation continued. Louise even resorted to giving herself enemas, a practice that I do not recommend because it can have serious side effects, such as increasing spasms, causing inflammation, or promoting a rectal ulcer.

I asked her to discontinue the enemas but to continue eating a high-fiber diet supplemented with psyllium fiber. I suggested that she make sure that she was walking briskly for a full thirty minutes each day.

Ultimately, I decided it was necessary to have Louise take a mild prescription laxative (such as Chronulac® syrup, a lactulose solution) to help alleviate her constipation and to ensure that she would not resort to taking any more enemas, which I consider a dangerous practice.

Medicines for Gas

As I stated earlier, for patients who are having trouble with gas I sometimes recommend activated charcoal tablets (Charcocaps), which provide relief from gas in the colon. I sometimes also recommend an over-the-counter preparation called Gas-X®, which contains simethicone, a foaming agent that joins small gas bubbles in the stomach into larger gas bubbles so that they are more easily belched away. These agents have helped some of my patients relieve gas, bloating, and cramps. But for the majority of my patients, I find that avoiding gas-producing foods, carbonated beverages, and gum and mints (which promote the swallowing of air) are sufficient to reduce gassy symptoms.

For those patients whose food journals indicate they have trouble digesting dairy products, I recommend the enzyme lactase (Lactaid®), available over-the-counter, which can be added to milk before drinking it. This enzyme can also be taken in tablet form just before eating foods such as cheese or ice cream that contain milk or milk products.

For my patients who have trouble digesting the sugar in beans and many vegetables, I sometimes recommend a nonprescription digestive aid called Beano®. Several drops of this enzyme added to beans or vegetables just before serving breaks down the gas-producing sugar.

Sometimes Even Doctors Have Trouble Deciding If Medicines Are Needed

The decision to use common-sense lifestyle approaches to treat GI distress is not difficult. The decision whether to use drugs or alternative medicines is more difficult—it is one of the gray areas of medicine. Thus, a healthy diet, aerobic exercise, avoidance of alcohol and tobacco, and other lifestyle modifications are clear-cut recommendations. Difficulties arise when we must go beyond common sense. Most drugs are not 100 percent effective, but they are effective more often than not. However, most drugs carry with them side effects, some of which are significant and may occur in at least 2 percent of people.

What About Alternative Medicines?

Many of my patients come to me asking about the use of some herb or potion that they have heard about. Often the agent in question has been recommended to them by a well-meaning family member who read about it in a magazine article or was told through the grapevine that it "did wonders" for someone's cousin. Some patients think that herbal teas such as chamomile "calm" their stomach. Chamomile tea is safe but not necessarily helpful. Other patients are convinced that herbal laxatives "cleanse" their system, allowing them to have regular bowel movements. In general, the active ingredient in such laxatives is no different than the active ingredient in traditional medicines found at the drugstore—and in some cases, that same ingredient can be found in foods. For example, some herbal laxatives contain senna, the same compound that is the active ingredient in over-the-counter drugs such as Senokot®—and which is found in prunes and prune juice. However, since the dosages in alternative preparations are often not indicated, you can easily take too much of them.

> *QUESTION "NATURAL"*
> Remember that just because a treatment is "natural" doesn't mean that it is safe and without side effects. Many "natural" herbal remedies can cause serious side effects in some people and can also cause problems if taken in conjunction with a prescription drug. Always check with your doctor before trying any herbal medicine.

I tell my patients that most alternative medicines are unproven. Although the impression may exist among users that alternative medicines are helpful, they have not been subjected to rigorous scientific evaluation as regular drugs have. Well-designed studies to eliminate the possibilities of misinterpretation of results or to properly evaluate the short- and long-term safety of medicines are usually lacking with alternative medicines. They are not regulated by the Food and Drug Administration (FDA), and therefore there may be variations in the contents of alternative medicines when multiple extracts, herbs, and other agents are combined in a single product. The relative concentrations of the various ingredients may vary because the FDA is not regulating its production processes. Furthermore, the safety of the contents of alternative medicines is not always carefully established.

Thus, once we have gone beyond the need for common-sense lifestyle modifications, it is essential that patients and physicians use careful judgment to assess whether or not the use of medicines (either FDA-approved ones or alternative ones) is appropriate. Since each individual patient is a unique, complex being, many factors must be carefully weighed. An experienced physician can look at the patient's lifestyle, personality, symptoms, and disease severity, and can weigh them against the available treatment options. This evaluation process cannot be adequately performed by a computer. It requires a thinking physician who can make an informed judgment and, from that, make a recommendation to the patient.

As an example, let me tell you about a thirty-four-year-old woman who had moderate irritable bowel syndrome for many years. During the past one and a half years, she had experienced the onset of progressive fatigue (extreme tiredness). She consulted several physicians who performed a variety of tests, but were unable to find a reasonable explanation for her fatigue. Finally, one doctor suggested that she must have chronic fatigue syndrome, a condition in which the person is infected with a virus called the Epstein-Barr virus. The physician performed blood tests that showed that she had an antibody to the Epstein-Barr virus.

In the mind of the patient, this test proved that she had chronic fatigue syndrome. However, neither the patient nor the physician realized that about one in every four people in Southern California have an antibody to the Epstein-Barr virus, and that its presence does not necessarily indicate the presence of infection.

In fact, it is the kind of antibody that reflects prior exposure to the virus, which is common in many parts of our country, but does not reflect ongoing infection. The physician offered the patient a variety of treatments for her "Epstein-Barr virus infection" but none were effective in relieving her fatigue. In desperation, the patient finally went to a Chinese herbalist who provided her with a variety of herbal preparations that he said would undoubtedly relieve her fatigue. The patient took the herbs and thought she even might be feeling less tired. Then her fatigue came back even more severely than in the past, and she developed yellow skin and eyes.

She was referred to me and it was clear that she had an acute form of toxic hepatitis that can result from some Chinese herbal medicines. I had her stop taking the Chinese herbs and her condition improved, but the fatigue did not totally go away. It was at this time that we undertook thyroid function studies and found that she was hypothyroid. She was given thyroid medication and, within two weeks, she started to improve. Her fatigue is now gone. Her liver tests are normal. She continues to have a mild to moderate intermittent irritable bowel syndrome. It was clear that what this patient needed was the guidance and judgment of an experienced physician. She needed the right drug at the right time, in this case thyroid medicine, but the desperate use of unproven treatments in this patient's situation led only to more serious problems.

Serious Gastrointestinal Disorders

There are certain conditions for which there is no doubt that drug treatment should be the first line of management and should not be delayed—even though common-sense approaches such as diet, exercise, and stress reduction techniques can be used to supplement them. Here are a few examples of more serious digestive conditions that have some of the same symptoms (such as abdominal pain, diarrhea, gas, and bloating) we have been discussing, but for which medications are almost always warranted.

Peptic Ulcers

Peptic ulcers are open sores or raw areas in the lining of the stomach (these are called gastric ulcers) or the beginning of the small intestine (these are called duodenal ulcers). People who have peptic ulcers experience a burning pain or a dull, gnawing pain in the affected area, usually below the rib cage, that comes and goes for several days or weeks. The pain often occurs in the middle of the night or several hours after meals, when the stomach is empty. Eating often relieves the pain quickly because food helps neutralize the acid in the stomach, but certain foods can produce more pain. Nearly one in every ten Americans develops an ulcer at some time in his or her life.

The most important thing to point out, however, is that peptic ulcers are *not* caused by spicy food or stress, as everyone—including doctors and scientists—had believed for over a hundred years. Doctors used to be taught that ulcers were psychosomatic and in large part related to tension, anxiety, and unhappiness. These emotional disturbances were thought to produce acid, which was thought to cause ulcers. That's why doctors used to recommend a bland diet and stress reduction for ulcers.

We now know that medicines (specifically antibiotics)—instead of just lifestyle modifications, such as diet changes and stress reduction—are needed to successfully treat most peptic ulcers. Research conducted around the world has revealed that most peptic ulcers are caused by infection with a bacteria called *Helicobacter pylori,* or *H. pylori* for short. *H. pylori* is diagnosed with a blood or breath test. (Some ulcers are caused by long-term use of nonsteroidal anti-inflammatory agents, called NSAIDs, like ibuprofen.) *H. pylori* weakens the protective mucous coating of the digestive tract, allowing acid to get through to the sensitive lining beneath. Both the acid and the bacteria irritate the lining and cause a sore, or ulcer. Lots of people are infected with *H. pylori,* but only some of these people develop ulcers. Scientists haven't yet figured out why.

In 1994, The National Institutes of Health (NIH) recommended treating *H. pylori* to cure peptic ulcers in those patients infected with the bacteria. The treatment regimen recommended by NIH is called the triple therapy: taking two antibiotics to kill the bacteria and an acid-suppressing drug for a period of two full weeks. This two-week regimen therapy reduces ulcer symptoms, kills the bacteria, and prevents ulcer recurrence in more than 90 percent of patients. Unfortunately, the antibiotics used in this therapy may cause mild side effects such as nausea, vomiting, diarrhea, metallic taste in the mouth, dizziness, headache, or yeast infections in women, but these side effects usually go away once the treatment is over.

Michael, a thirty-three-year-old businessman, was a patient of mine who thought dietary changes were needed to manage his symptoms, but who needed medicine instead. Michael came to me after having experienced five months of progressively increasing episodes of pain in the pit of his stomach. The pain usually came on after meals and had gradually increased in frequency and severity. In order to relieve the pain, he found himself frequently taking aspirin. He also tried taking antacids.

Michael was "too busy" to see a doctor, but he decided on his own that he probably had an ulcer since, as he put it, everyone knows that stress causes ulcers. After all, people were always saying, "This job is going to give me an ulcer!"

To treat his ulcer, Michael placed himself on a bland diet. He found that milk relieved his symptoms for a short period of time, so he got into the habit of drinking milk throughout the day. And, because he believed that stress was the cause of his ulcer, he tried to relieve his tension and anxiety by drinking wine or beer at the end of the day.

Nevertheless, his pain got worse, so eventually he found the time to come to see me.

In order to establish the basis of his diagnosis I had him undergo a test called an upper endoscopy. The test showed that he had a typical duodenal ulcer but he also had an inflammation of the lining of the stomach (a condition called gastritis), clearly due to the aspirin that he had been taking on a regular basis to relieve his pain. He also had an inflammation of the lining of the esophagus (a condition called esophagitis), which, I believe, was aggravated by his ingestion of alcohol, as was his gastritis. We took a biopsy of Michael's duodenal ulcer and found that, as expected, he was infected with *H. pylori*.

If you have a peptic ulcer, you may find that foods that increase the amount of acid in your stomach may worsen your stomach pain. Therefore, until your stomach heals, you may find it helpful to avoid acidic foods—such as citrus fruits and juices—and acid-producing foods, such as caffeine-containing foods and drinks and coffee (even the decaffeinated kind). In the same way, although stress doesn't cause ulcers, your stomach can produce extra acid when you're under stress, making your stomach pain worse. So, while you're taking your antibiotic and your stomach is healing, you'll feel better if you manage stressful situations appropriately, alleviating as much stress and anxiety as possible. (See chapter 5 for a detailed discussion of stress management.)

I treated Michael with a standard fourteen-day regimen of acid-reducing drugs together with two antibiotics to kill the *H. pylori*. Within that period of time his symptoms disappeared and did not subsequently recur.

In Michael's case, making lifestyle changes alone wouldn't have taken care of his gastrointestinal problem. Michael clearly needed medicine. In many, many other cases, however, patients who come to see me don't really need a prescription for medicines—they need a prescription for lifestyle modifications.

ULCER MYTH

Forget what you used to "know" about ulcers. They are not caused by stress or spicy food. Most ulcers are caused by a bacterial infection, and they can be cured by taking antibiotics. While the ulcer is healing, however, you may feel better if you avoid spicy foods, alcohol, and other foods that increase the amount of acid in your injured stomach.

Diverticulosis and Diverticulitis

Diverticulosis is a condition in which sacs (called diverticula) have formed in the walls of the intestines. People usually don't have any symptoms with diverticulosis. Diverticulitis is the name given to the condition when the sacs have become infected and inflamed, causing fever and lower abdominal pain and tenderness. Diverticulitis may also result in abscesses (infected areas of pus), bowel blockage, or breaks and leaks through the bowel wall.

Diverticulitis can sometimes cause serious problems. For instance, when one of the sacs becomes infected and inflamed, bacteria can enter small tears in the surface of the bowel, causing small abscesses. Such an infection may remain localized and go away within a few days. In rare cases, however, the infection spreads and breaks through the wall of the colon causing peritonitis—infection of the abdominal cavity—or abscesses in the abdomen. Such infections are extremely serious and must be treated without delay.

Most people recover from diverticulitis without surgery, but they do need to take antibiotics. Sometimes, however, people need surgery to drain an abscess that has resulted from a ruptured sac (diverticulum) and to remove that portion of the colon. Recommendations for surgery are usually reserved for individuals with severe or multiple attacks.

Let's look at an example of a patient who had diverticulitis. Ted was a sixty-seven-year-old retired engineer who had been coming to my office for many years because of his irritable bowel syndrome. Recently, however, he had begun waking up at night with diarrhea and severe cramping in the left lower part of his abdomen. The next day he had fever and chills and his diarrhea continued and his pain worsened. The left lower part of his abdomen was tender when it was touched. He presumed that these symptoms were an unusual attack of his irritable bowel syndrome.

When I examined him, it was clear to me that the inflammation of Ted's abdomen indicated that he had diverticulitis. His tender abdomen and his elevated temperature suggested that a pocket in the wall of the bowel had become obstructed and infected, and that a small pocket of pus surrounded by inflamed tissue had developed. There was no doubt that Ted required antibiotic treatment if we were going to avoid emergency surgery. Ted began taking the antibiotic I prescribed for him, and within twenty-four hours his fever disappeared and his pain lessened. His diarrhea soon came under better control, and within three days he was feeling well. I told Ted that it was crucial that he take the full ten-day course of antibiotics he was given, and that he not stop taking them just because his symptoms had abated. I explained to him that if his symptoms recurred, we might have to consider surgically removing part of his intestine.

This was a situation in which a patient who had underlying irritable bowel syndrome developed a second disease. The patient could not make the judgment as to whether this was a new or different illness, but as an experienced physician, I could easily tell by examining him that a new and potentially serious condition had developed, one that required immediate treatment with medication, in this case antibiotics. There was no doubt that drug treatment was appropriate here—and lifestyle modification measures would have not been able to solve Ted's problem.

Ulcerative Colitis

Ulcerative colitis is a condition in which parts of the large intestine become inflamed causing abdominal cramps, diarrhea, and often rectal bleeding. Joint pain and skin sores or rashes may also develop. Ulcerative colitis is an inflammatory bowel disease (IBD), the general name for diseases that cause inflammation in the intestines. Ulcerative colitis can be difficult to diagnose because its symptoms are similar to other intestinal disorders such as irritable bowel syndrome and to another type of IBD called Crohn's disease (see below). Crohn's disease differs from ulcerative colitis because it causes inflammation deeper within the intestinal wall, and Crohn's disease often occurs in the small intestine, but it can also occur in the mouth, esophagus, stomach, duodenum, large intestine, appendix, and anus.

Treatment for ulcerative colitis depends on the seriousness of the disease. Most cases are treated with medication to suppress the inflammatory process, permit healing of the intestine, and relieve the diarrhea, rectal bleeding, and abdominal cramps.

A patient who had ulcerative colitis was a twenty-seven-year-old woman named Julia who had been having two or three attacks of bloody diarrhea each year for the past three years. She went to see her family doctor, who referred her to me. I performed a test called a colonoscopy, which showed inflammation and ulcerations of Julia's colon. I prescribed a medicine called Asacol® (5-aminosalicylic acid), and she did pretty well taking it. However, a few weeks later, Julia's job became especially stressful, and she found that her bloody diarrhea had come back. She was having as many as fifteen bloody loose stools within a twenty-four-hour period, and was having to get up in the middle of the night because of it. She came to see me and I found that she had a fever of 101° F. I then prescribed another drug, an oral corticosteroid called prednisone. Over the following few days, her diarrhea became less frequent until she was only experiencing one or two stools per day, and they were no longer bloody. Over time, I weaned her off the prednisone, and she continued to do well.

Julia's condition was so severe that it required medication, but once her diarrhea was under control, I recommended that Julia read about the relaxation response and that she practice meditation techniques to help her manage stress, with the goal of helping her learn to manage her ulcerative colitis in the future.

Crohn's Disease

Crohn's disease is an inflammatory condition that may affect any part of the gastrointestinal tract from the mouth to the anus. However, it mainly involves the lower part of the small intestine (called the ileum) and the large intestine (colon).

Symptoms of Crohn's disease usually include diarrhea and crampy abdominal pain following a meal, and they may also include fever, fatigue, and rectal bleeding. Loss of appetite and subsequent weight loss may also occur. Other symptoms can include sores in the anal area, fissures (cracks), fistulas (abnormal openings connecting the bowel to the skin surface near the anus), and abscesses (sacs filled with pus). These symptoms may range from mild to severe.

Because Crohn's disease is similar to ulcerative colitis, the two disorders are grouped together as inflammatory bowel disease (IBD). Because no medical cure for Crohn's disease exists, the goals of medical treatment are to suppress the inflammatory response, permit healing of tissue, and relieve the symptoms of fever, diarrhea, and abdominal pain.

Good nutrition is important in the management of Crohn's disease to restore fluids and nutrients that are lost because of reduced appetite and diarrhea. And, while symptoms are flaring, soft, bland foods may cause less discomfort than spicy or high-fiber foods.

As with many other gastrointestinal disorders, stress can influence the course of Crohn's disease, and stress-reducing techniques can help manage symptoms.

Smoking has been shown to worsen the symptoms of Crohn's disease, and I always insist that my Crohn's disease patients who smoke take steps (such as using a nicotine patch) as soon as possible to quit smoking.

One of my patients, mentioned in chapter 2, had been smoking for nearly thirty years, and his nicotine habit contributed greatly to the severe abdominal pain, diarrhea, and cramping he experienced due to Crohn's disease. As the years went by, his Crohn's disease worsened. He developed fistulas, which are spontaneous connections between loops of bowel or between loops of bowel and the skin. These were associated with drainage of fecal material. He developed abscesses (pockets of pus) within the abdomen and signs of intestinal blockage, so it was necessary that we perform a series of surgical procedures in which segments of his intestine were removed. With each operation, he would quit smoking, resolving never to start again. But once the crisis was over, his nicotine habit would return.

For this man, making the lifestyle change to quit smoking was extremely difficult. So, for him, not only medication but surgery was necessary. Had he been able to quit smoking before too much damage was done, he may have avoided the surgery.

One of my patients, a forty-year-old woman, had had Crohn's disease for more than twenty years. Her flares of diarrhea, cramping, and abdominal pain, often associated with fever and weight loss, had initially been treated with short courses of prednisone (cortisone). In order to control her episodes, she could not be weaned off the prednisone, and eventually her short courses became a continuous course of daily prednisone administration. This had gone on for ten years and she had begun to experience the ravages of cortisone treatment. She developed cataracts, which eventually were treated surgically. She frequently got upper respiratory infections and experienced two episodes of pneumonia because she was more susceptible to infection, but recently she was devastated by the development of very severe pain in the right hip. On X-ray examination, she was found to have "aseptic necrosis" of the hip. This collapse of the bone is a clear-cut sign of long-term cortisone use. She then underwent a series of difficult operations in order to preserve her mobility and to relieve her pain. However, it was clear that the side effects of cortisone outweighed the benefits that the drug had for her underlying disease. She was placed on a low dose of 6-mercaptopurine (an immuno-suppressive drug, which may increase susceptibility to infection, but usually in higher doses). Since it takes three to six months for the beneficial effects of 6-mercaptopurine, she was given an antibiotic, Metronidazole, which has also been shown to have beneficial effects on many patients with Crohn's disease. After six months, the Metronidazole was stopped and she was maintained on 6-mercaptopurine. The drug was highly effective and greatly reduced the severity and frequency of her symptoms. Once she started to do well, we were able to taper and eventually discontinue her Prednisone. Essentially, we took her off a drug with devastating side effects, and substituted a step-down drug that was effective and had less severe side effects.

Pancreatitis

Pancreatitis is an inflammation of the pancreas, the large gland behind the stomach that secretes digestive juices into the first part of the small intestine (duodenum) and insulin into the bloodstream. In acute pancreatitis, some of the digestive juices—which contain digestive enzymes—escape from the ducts of the pancreas, where they are supposed to be and cause no harm, and into the tissue of the pancreas itself. There, the digestive enzymes cause severe acute damage to the pancreas and surrounding tissues and can even lead to bleeding in the pancreas. Pancreatitis sometimes occurs spontaneously, but sometimes it occurs in association with factors such as physical injury to the upper abdomen, gallbladder disease, or alcohol abuse.

Treatment depends upon the seriousness of the problem and possible underlying factors. In chronic cases of pancreatitis, in which the function of the pancreas has been impaired, oral medication is used to replace digestive enzymes.

To illustrate what can happen when one has pancreatitis, let me tell you about Frank, a fifty-seven-year-old man who had a long history—more than twenty years—of alcohol abuse. About five years ago, Frank started having recurring episodes of nausea, vomiting, and pain in his abdomen. He also had diarrhea with loose, greasy stools that were yellowish and floated in the toilet, leaving an oily ring around the toilet bowl.

Frank went to his doctor, who performed laboratory tests and found that his blood levels of certain enzymes (called amylase and lipase) were too high. His abdomen was tender and he was running a fever. Because of these signs and Frank's history of alcohol abuse, his doctor diagnosed his condition as alcoholic pancreatitis. Frank began to lose a lot of weight even though he was eating a reasonable diet, so he was hospitalized temporarily and fed intravenously (through a tube in his vein).

When he returned home, he continued to lose weight,

and within a year he had lost a total of fifty pounds. He was referred to me and I advised him to avoid all alcohol, which he did—with the help of Alcoholics Anonymous. I prescribed pancreatic enzyme supplements, because his body was no longer producing enough of these pancreatic enzymes on its own.

His stools returned to a normal color and were no longer greasy. He regained much of the weight that he lost, and he continues feeling better to this day. Clearly, Frank could have avoided his pancreatitis if he had avoided alcohol much earlier, but, by the time he came to see me, his condition was so severe that he required medication.

In this book, I have shown you that in many cases, people with heartburn, gas, bloating, diarrhea, and constipation can relieve their symptoms through diet and lifestyle changes—without using medicines, but that there are other times when medicines are needed. Deciding whether your particular case warrants use of medicines is best left up to a qualified doctor. Once your doctor has ruled out serious complications and has agreed that lifestyle modifications are a good way to manage your particular condition, you can use the strategies outlined in this book to determine your own best plan of attack.

Even if your doctor believes that medicines are needed to bring your condition under control, he or she will likely agree that lifestyle modifications like those discussed in this book would be a helpful addition to your treatment plan. Eventually (depending on the kind of disorder you have), you may be able to limit or even discontinue your medication and manage your condition with a healthful diet, exercise program, and stress management.

RESOURCES

··

Recommended Reading

Chapter 1

Be Good to Your Gut: Recipes and Tips for People with Digestive Problems by Pat Baird, R.D. (Blackwell Science, 1996), offers practical tips and recipes from a registered dietitian.

Eating Right for a Bad Gut: The Complete Nutritional Guide to Ileitis, Colitis, Crohn's Disease, and Inflammatory Bowel Disease by Dr. James Scala (Plume, 1992), discusses dietary changes to relieve the symptoms of digestive diseases.

Gastrointestinal Health: A Self-Help Nutritional Program to Prevent, Cure, or Alleviate Irritable Bowel Syndrome, Ulcers, Heartburn, Gas, Constipation by Steven R. Peikin (HarperCollins, 1991), provides lifestyle tips for managing digestive disorders.

Heartburn and What to Do About It by Dr. James F. Balch and Dr. Morton Walker (Avery Publishing Group, 1998), discusses drug-free ways to manage gastrointestinal discomforts.

Irritable Bowel Syndrome and the Mind-Body Brain-Gut Connection by William B. Salt II, M.D. (Parkview Publishing, 1997), offers practical suggestions for managing gastrointestinal disorders through lifestyle changes.

The Gastrointestinal Sourcebook by M. Sara Rosenthal (Lowell House, 1999). Provides a complete overview of the entire digestive process and includes information on symptoms, treatments, and management techniques for conditions from ulcers and gastroesophageal reflux to IBS and other upper and lower gastrointestinal disorders.

Wind Breaks: Coming to Terms with Wind by gastroenterologist Terry Bolin and nutritionist Rosemary Stanton (Margaret Gee Publishing, Double Bay NSW, Australia, 1993), discusses in detail the biochemistry of gas production, and suggests ways to manage excess gas, including the use of activated charcoal and avoiding gas-producing foods.

Chapter 2

Relief from IBS by Elaine Fantle Shimberg (Ballantine Books, 1988) is an easy-to-read paperback by a patient who has firsthand experience with the symptoms of irritable bowel syndrome. Readers get an inside look at life with irritable bowel syndrome, and how diet, exercise, and stress relief can help.

Seven Weeks to a Settled Stomach by Ronald L. Hoffman, M.D. (Pocket Books, 1990), offers practical recommendations for making lifestyle changes that can lead to better digestive health.

Stomach Ailments and Digestive Disturbances by Michael T. Murray (The Getting Well Naturally Series, Prima Publishing, 1997). Provides practical information and sensible advice for getting and staying well naturally.

The Healthy Heart Walking Book: The American Heart Association Walking Program by The American Heart Association (IDG Books Worldwide, 1995). Outlines a walking program designed to improve cardiovascular health, and offers advice for getting started and building endurance.

The Wellness Book: The Comprehensive Guide to Maintaining Health and Treating Stress-Related Illness by Herbert Benson, M.D. and Eileen M. Stuart, R.N., M.S. (Simon & Schuster, 1992), provides in-depth discussions of how mind/body medicine can be used to treat illnesses.

Chapter 3

American Heart Association has several excellent cookbooks, including *AHA Low-Fat, Low-Cholesterol Cookbook: Heart-Healthy, Easy-to-Make Recipes That Taste Great* (2d ed.), *AHA Quick and Easy Cookbook: Over 200 Healthful Recipes You Can Prepare in Minutes, AHA Meals in Minutes: More Low-Fat, Quick and Easy Recipes,* and *The New American Heart Association Cookbook, 25th Anniversary Edition.* All books published by Times Books/ Clarkson Potter.

American Medical Association's Family Cookbook by Melanie Barnard and Brooke Dojny with Mindy Hermann, R.D., and C. Wayne Callaway, M.D. (Pocket Books, 1999), offers low-fat cooking tips and recipes that are easy to follow.

The Essential Guide to Nutrition and the Foods We Eat by Jean

Pennington, Ph.D., R.D. (American Dietetic Association, 1999), provides tables of the nutritional values for many foods—including portion sizes and fat content.

Portion Savvy: The 30-Day Smart Plan for Eating Well by Carrie Latt (Pocket Books, 1999), includes a "pop-out" centerfold of sturdy paper food-portion guides to help you eyeball right-size servings.

Prevention magazine's food editors also have a cookbook called *The Healthy Cook: The Ultimate Illustrated Kitchen Guide to Great Low-Fat Food* (Rodale Press, 1997).

Chapter 4

Fitting in Fitness by American Heart Association (Times Books/Crown Publishing Group, 1998) has hundreds of tips to help you squeeze in exercise when you have no time to exercise.

Real-World Fitness by Kathy Kaehler, fitness consultant to the *Today* show (Golden Books, 1999), includes a chapter called "Stealth Fitness: Sneaking More Activity into Your Daily Life."

Smart Guide to Getting Strong and Fit by Carole Bodgers (John Wiley & Sons, 1998), gives advice on starting an exercise program.

Walking: A Complete Guide to the Complete Exercise by Casey Meyers (Random House, 1992), provides all you need to know about starting a walking program, including an excellent discussion of the benefits of walking.

Chapter 5

American Cancer Society's Freshstart: 21 Days to Stop Smoking by Dee Burton, Ph.D. (Pocket Books, 1986). This is a step-by-step approach that gets people through the first three weeks of smoking cessation, explaining what is happening along the way.

American Lung Association 7 Steps to a Smoke-Free Life by the American Lung Association; Edwin B. Fisher, Jr., and C. Everett Koop (John Wiley & Sons, 1998). Based on the American Lung Association's "Freedom from Smoking" program, the book emphasizes finding the reasons one smokes and identifying your personal triggers. The book is interactively organized, presenting information that helps you understand your habit and break it, worksheets, and checklists to personalize your plan.

Lifeskills by Virginia and Redford Williams (Crown Publishers, 1998), offers easy-to-follow guidelines for reducing stress through more effective communication.

New Yoga Challenge by the American Yoga Association with Alice Christensen (Contemporary Books, 1996), provides powerful workouts for flexibility, strength, energy, and inner discovery.

Quit Smart: Stop Smoking with the Quit Smart System by Robert H. Shipley (JB Press, 1999). Based on the premise that successful quitting is not so much a matter of willpower as it is a skill of doing the right things and thinking the right thoughts to succeed, the book also presents up-to-date information on many issues facing a person trying to quit smoking.

Quit Smoking for Good: A Supportive Program for Permanent Smoking Cessation by Andre Baer (Crossing Press, 1998). Provides emotional and behavioral preparation for life without cigarettes.

Stress, Diet, and Your Heart by Dean Ornish, M.D. (New

American Library, 1984), presents several powerful stress-reduction techniques, including progressive deep relaxation, breathing techniques, and meditation.

Stress Management: A Comprehensive Guide to Wellness by Edward Charlesworth, Ph.D. and Ronald Nathan, Ph.D. (Ballantine Books, 1982), is from the American Academy of Behavioral Medicine and offers a wide spectrum of stress-reducing strategies.

The Enlightened Smoker's Guide to Quitting by B. Jack Gebhardt (Element, 1998). Presents a seven-step program to quit smoking. Gebhardt uses this program in seminars including one for the American Cancer Society.

The Relaxation and Stress Reduction Workbook by Martha Davis, Ph.D., Elizabeth Robbins Eshelman, M.S.W., and Matthew McKay, Ph.D. (New Harbinger Publications, Inc., Fourth Edition, 1995), provides step-by-step directions for a host of stress-reduction techniques.

The Relaxation Response by Herbert Benson, M.D. (Avon Books, 1975), a classic work that defines and describes how to elicit the relaxation response, a simple meditative technique that's still widely used today to manage stress.

The Stop Smoking Workbook by Lori Stevic-Rust (Contributor) and Anita Maximin (New Harbinger Publishing, 1996). Uses practical exercises to help smokers understand the realities of addiction and the stages of quitting.

20-Minute Yoga Workouts by the American Yoga Association with Alice Christensen (Ballantine Books, 1995), provides simple but powerful exercises to reach everyone who takes a few minutes a day to practice this technique.

You Can Stop Smoking by Jacquelyn Rogers and Julie Rubenstein (Pocket Books, 1995). Jacquelyn Rogers, a former two-pack a day smoker, shares facts and tips through her SmokEnders program.

Chapter 6

Heartburn: Extinguishing the Fire Inside by M. Michael Wolfe, M.D., and Thomas Nesi (W. W. Norton, 1997), explains the advantages of H_2 blockers, points out the dangers of overusing antacids, and discusses the use of lifestyle modifications to manage heartburn.

"Irritable Bowel Syndrome," by Bernard Coulie, M.D., Ph.D., and Michael Camilleri, M.D., in the medical journal *Clinical Perspectives in Gastroenterology*, November/ December 1999, pp. 329–38. This article, written for physicians, provides in-depth information about the treatment of irritable bowel syndrome.

The Second Brain: A Groundbreaking New Understanding of Nervous Disorders of the Stomach and Intestine by Michael D. Gershon, M.D. (HarperPerennial Library, 1999). Offers groundbreaking research revealing that a "second brain" in the abdomen must cooperate with the main brain to insure gastrointestinal health.

Ulcers: A Guide to Diagnosis, Treatment, and Prevention by Ricki Ostrov (Thorsons Publishing, 1996). Defines ulcers and the bacteria that causes them, and provides information on the digestive tract, diagnosis, treatment, and prevention.

Helpful Organizations

Aerobics and Fitness Association of America
800-225-2322
www.afaa.com

American College of Gastroenterology
4900 B South 31st Street
Arlington, VA 22206
(703) 820-7400
(703) 931-4520 fax
(800) HRT-BURN (487-2876)
www.acg.gi.org/patientinfo/frame_gerd.html

American College of Sports Medicine
P.O. Box 1440
Indianapolis, IN 46206
800-486-5643
www.acsm.org

American Council on Exercise
5820 Oberlin Drive, Suite 102
San Diego, CA 92121
800-529-8227
www.acefitness.org

American Dietetic Association
National Center for Nutrition and Dietetics
216 West Jackson Blvd.
Chicago, IL 60606
800-366-1655 (Consumer Nutrition Hot Line)

www.eatright.org
Provides healthy lifestyle tips and information about nutrition, as well as referrals to registered dietitians.

American Heart Association
7272 Greenville Ave.
Dallas, TX 75231
800-AHA-USA1 (800-242-8721)
www.americanheart.org
This site provides excellent information about nutrition and exercise.

American Yoga Association
P.O. Box 19986
Sarasota, FL 34276-2986
(941) 927-4977
http://members.aol.com/amyogaassn

National Digestive Diseases Information Clearinghouse
2 Information Way
Bethesda, MD 20892-3570
(301) 654-3810
www.niddk.nih.gov
Fact sheets are available on a variety of digestive diseases including: "Your Digestive System and How It Works," "Gastroesophageal Reflux Disease," "Constipation," and "Irritable Bowel Syndrome."

National Institute of Diabetes and Digestive and Kidney Diseases
1 WIN Way

Bethesda, MD 20892-3665
(800) WIN-8098
(301) 984-7196 fax
www.niddk.nih.gov/health/nutrit/win.htm
This government agency provides fact sheets, brochures, video-taped lectures on topics concerning nutrition and weight control, as well as a newsletter and links to other weight-control Web sites.

Shape Up America!
6707 Democracy Blvd., Suite 306
Bethesda, MD 20817
301-493-5368
www.shapeup.org
Shape Up America! was founded by former U.S. Surgeon-General C. Everett Koop. The Shape Up America! Web site provides helpful information about healthy eating and increasing physical activity. It also offers practical solutions to problems like unsupportive family members and foods that promote binge eating. Links are also provided to message boards and support networks.

The American Lung Association
1740 Broadway
New York, NY 10019
(212) 315-8700
www.lungusa.org

www.arhp.org/clinical/clinical1. This site from The Association of Reproductive Health Professionals is geared toward scientific information available to the public. The site contains information from smoking and premature aging to smoking cessation programs for pregnant women. Although the site does not have information about how to stop smoking, there is a lot of information including how to reach young people before they begin to smoke.

www.cancer.org. Once on this site from The American Cancer Society, go under "Tobacco Control" for more in-depth information on the following: health issues (youth tobacco use, cigar smoking, clear indoor air, and so on), quitting tips (including their programs and smokeless tobacco), public issues, and finally smoking-related cancers. Furthermore, the site contains their smoking cessation program called "Freshstart" which consists of four one-hour sessions. A very informative Web site. I highly recommend it.

www.smokenders.com. Smokenders is a twenty-nine-year-old program that allows participants to continue to smoke until the last two weeks of the seven-week program, making it seem less threatening than other smoking cessation programs. It also has a toll-free support line.

INDEX

....

Italicized page numbers refer to drawings.

ABOUT THE AUTHOR

....

Gary Gitnick, M.D., is Professor of Medicine and Chief of the Division of Digestive Diseases at the University of California, Los Angeles School of Medicine, the largest gastroenterology division in the world. With more than 30 years of experience, he has written more than 300 publications and is the author or editor of 63 books on digestive distress. He resides in Encino, California.